HANDBOOK *of*
RETINAL**OCT**

Content Strategist: *Russell Gabbedy*
Content Development Specialist: *Sharon Nash*
Project Manager: *Julie Taylor*
Design: *Christian Bilbow*
Illustration Manager: *Jennifer Rose*
Illustrator: *Antbits Ltd*
Marketing Manager(s) (UK/USA): *Gaynor Jones/Abby Swartz*

HANDBOOK *of* RETINAL **OCT**

Lead Editor

Jay S. Duker MD
Director, New England Eye Center
Professor and Chairman,
   Department of Ophthalmology
Tufts Medical Center
Tufts University School of Medicine
Boston, MA, USA

Associate Editors

Nadia K. Waheed MD MPH
Assistant Professor of Ophthalmology
New England Eye Center
Tufts Medical Center
Tufts University School of Medicine
Boston, MA, USA

Darin R. Goldman MD
Vitreoretinal Surgeon
Retina Group of Florida
Fort Lauderdale, FL, USA

For additional online content visit
expertconsult

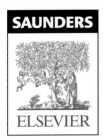

London, New York, Oxford, Philadelphia, St Louis, Sydney, Toronto

ELSEVIER
SAUNDERS

Notices

Knowledge and best practice in this field are constantly changing. As new research and experience broaden our understanding, changes in research methods, professional practices, or medical treatment may become necessary.

Practitioners and researchers must always rely on their own experience and knowledge in evaluating and using any information, methods, compounds, or experiments described herein. In using such information or methods they should be mindful of their own safety and the safety of others, including parties for whom they have a professional responsibility.

With respect to any drug or pharmaceutical products identified, readers are advised to check the most current information provided (i) on procedures featured or (ii) by the manufacturer of each product to be administered, to verify the recommended dose or formula, the method and duration of administration, and contraindications. It is the responsibility of practitioners, relying on their own experience and knowledge of their patients, to make diagnoses, to determine dosages and the best treatment for each individual patient, and to take all appropriate safety precautions.

To the fullest extent of the law, neither the Publisher nor the authors, contributors, or editors, assume any liability for any injury and/or damage to persons or property as a matter of products liability, negligence or otherwise, or from any use or operation of any methods, products, instructions, or ideas contained in the material herein.

ISBN: 978-0-323-18884-5
e-book ISBN: 978-0-323-18885-2

your source for books,
journals and multimedia
in the health sciences

www.elsevierhealth.com

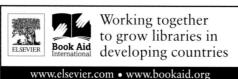

Working together
to grow libraries in
developing countries

www.elsevier.com • www.bookaid.org

The publisher's policy is to use paper manufactured from sustainable forests

Printed in China
Last digit is the print number: 9 8 7 6 5 4 3 2 1

Contents

Contents

Contents

Preface

Optical coherence tomography (OCT) was 'discovered' in an optics lab at the Massachusetts Institute of Technology in the late 1980s by James Fujimoto and his collaborators: Carmen Puliafito, Joel Schuman, David Huang, Eric Swanson and Mike Hee. It began as an effort to experimentally measure excimer laser corneal ablation in real time. While it failed in that regard, the founders quickly identified the possibility that OCT could be employed to measure static ocular tissue thickness in real time. The first publication on OCT was in *Science* in 1991 and by 1996 the technology was transferred to a commercial company and soon thereafter commercial devices began to be sold.

In 2013, it is safe to say that OCT is one of the most important ancillary tests in ophthalmology and it is indisputably THE most important ancillary test in the subspecialty of the retina. We set out to produce an easy-to-read, brief but complete handbook of OCT images that was disease-based. Given the importance of OCT in our practices, we concluded that the OCT images should be the major focus of the book. Consistency of chapter layout, excellent images, and well-documented pathologic features were all goals. This book has minimal clinical description of the pathologic entities. There are plenty of excellent textbooks that cover these entities in more depth. We hope you find this handbook useful in your clinical practice on a daily basis.

Daniela Ferrara MD PhD
Researcher
New England Eye Center
Tufts University School of Medicine
Boston, MA, USA

Sana Nadeem MBBS FCPS
Senior Registrar
Ophthalmology Department
Fauji Foundation Hospital
Rawalpindi, Pakistan

Alexandre S.C. Reis MD
Department of Ophthalmology
University of São Paulo
São Paulo, SP, Brazil

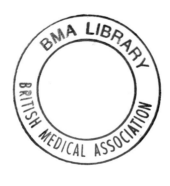

Acknowledgements

The development of optical coherence tomography and its emergence as the most important ancillary test in ophthalmology is inextricably linked to the New England Eye Center at Tufts Medical Center and its physicians. The clinical experiences summarized in this book are based on the collective expertise gained at the Eye Center over the past two decades and we are very grateful to our colleagues Caroline Baumal, Elias Reichel, Chris Robinson, Adam Rogers and Andre Witkin, with whom we are privileged to share patients and who have been an inexhaustible resource for this endeavor. We would also like to acknowledge the unparalleled ophthalmic imaging department at the New England Eye Center whose members acquired most of the images included in this book. Thanks also go out to the contributing authors and to our production team at Elsevier who worked on a very tight schedule to get the book published in just over six months. Our fellows and residents, whose questions provide constant intellectual challenge, also deserve acknowledgement. And last but perhaps most importantly, we would like to thank our families for their patience and support.

Dedications

To my wife Julie and my children, Jake, Bear, Sam and Elly whose support, love, patience and understanding allow me to pursue projects like this book. Also, to Carmen Puliafito, Joel Schuman and Jim Fujimoto – without them OCT would not exist and without their mentorship and collaboration I would never have been immersed in it.

Jay S. Duker

To Khadija and Ahmed, for their patience, generosity and encouragement. To my mother, the constant inspiration, without whom none of this would be possible. To my mentors past and present, and to my co-authors who made the process of writing this book such a phenomenally enjoyable and educational experience.

Nadia K. Waheed

To my wife Robin, whose constant love and encouragement allow me to pursue my passions, and to my parents Marisse and Tony and sister Candice, whose support I am forever grateful to have.

Darin Goldman

Glossary

AMD age-related macular degeneration
ARN acute retinal necrosis

BM Bruch's membrane
BRAO branch retinal artery occlusion
BRVO branch retinal vein occlusion

CiRAO cilioretinal artery occlusion
CME cystoid macular edema
CNV choroidal neovascularization
CRAO central retinal artery occlusion
CRVO central retinal vein occlusion
CSCR central serous chorioretinopathy
CWS cotton wool spots

DME diabetic macular edema
DR diabetic retinopathy

EDI enhanced depth imaging
ELM external limiting membrane
ERM epiretinal membrane
ETDRS Early Treatment of Diabetic
Retinopathy Study

FA fluorescein angiography
FAF fundus autofluorescence
FD Fourier domain
FTMH full-thickness macular hole

GA geographic atrophy
GCC ganglion cell complex

HE hard exudates
HRVO hemiretinal vein occlusion

ICGA indocyanine green angiography
ICP intracranial pressure
ILM internal limiting membrane
INL inner nuclear layer
IPL inner plexiform layer
IRF intraretinal fluid

IRMA intraretinal microvascular
abnormalities
IS inner segment of photoreceptors
IS–OS inner segment – outer segment
(of photoreceptors)

LE left eye
LMH lamellar macular hole

MacTel macular telangiectasia
MCP multifocal choroiditis with panuveitis

NFL nerve fiber layer
NPDR non-proliferative diabetic
retinopathy
NVD neovascularization of the disc
NVE neovascularization elsewhere (retinal
neovascularization)
NVI neovascularization of the iris

OCT optical coherence tomography
ONH optic nerve head
ONL outer nuclear layer
OPL outer plexiform layer
OS outer segment of photoreceptors

PCME postoperative cystoid macular
edema
PCV polypoidal choroidal vasculopathy
PDR proliferative diabetic retinopathy
PED pigment epithelial detachment
PFC perfluorocarbon
PVD posterior vitreous detachment

RAP retinal angiomatous proliferation
RCH retinal capillary hemangioma
RD retinal detachment
RE right eye
RNFL retinal nerve fiber layer
RP retinitis pigmentosa
RPE retinal pigment epithelium

RRD rhegmatogenous retinal detachment
RS retinoschisis

SD spectral domain
SD-OCT spectral domain optical coherence tomography
SRF subretinal fluid
SS swept source
SVP summed voxel projection

TD time domain
TD-OCT time domain optical coherence tomography

TRD tractional retinal detachment
TSINT temporal, superior, inferior, nasal temporal scan pattern

VEGF vascular endothelial growth factor
VKH Vogt–Koyanagi–Harada
VMA vitreomacular adhesion
VMT vitreomacular traction
VRL vitreoretinal lymphoma

XLRS X-linked juvenile retinoschisis

PART 1: Introduction to OCT

1.1 Scanning Principles

Optical coherence tomography (OCT) is a medical diagnostic imaging technology that captures micron resolution three-dimensional images. It is based on the principle of optical reflectometry, which involves the measurement of light back-scattering through transparent or semi-transparent media such as biological tissues. It achieves this by measuring the intensity and the echo time delay of light that is scattered from the tissues of interest. Light from a broadband light source is broken into two arms, a reference arm and a sample arm that is reflected back from structures at various depths within the posterior pole of the eye.

There are two main ways in which the backscattered light can be detected:

▸ Time domain (TD) detection
▸ Fourier domain (FD) detection – which is further broken down into:
  • Spectral domain (SD)
  • Swept source (SS)

Time Domain OCT

In time domain OCT scanning, light from the reference arm and light reflected back from the sample undergo interference, and the interference over time is used to generate an 'A-scan' depth resolved image of the retina at a single point. Moving the sample and the light source with respect to each other generates multiple A-scans that are combined into a cross-sectional linear image called the B-scan or 'line scan'. Scanning speeds of TD-OCTs are typically around 400 A-scans/second. The primary commercially available TD-OCT device is the Stratus OCT™ made by Carl Zeiss Meditech.

Spectral Domain OCT

In this technology, the spectral interference pattern between the reference beam and the sample beam is dispersed by a spectrometer and collected simultaneously with an array detector. This simultaneous collection allows for much faster scanning speeds than the traditional time domain devices where a mechanically moving interferometer gathers the data over time. An A-scan is then generated using an inverse Fourier transform on the simultaneously gathered data. Commercially available SD-OCT devices have scanning rates of 18,000–70,000 A-scans/second.

Higher scan speeds in the SD-OCT faster acquisition time, which minimizes the chance of eye movements during acquisition, especially in patients with poor fixation. Both hardware and software enhancements permit precise image registration which allows for more reliable comparison between visits. Faster acquisition speeds also mean a higher sampling density of the macula, minimizing the chances of missing pathology. The higher speeds allow for the production of three-dimensional OCT scans. The broader light sources of SD-OCT devices achieve a higher axial resolution than TD-OCT, allowing better visualization of retinal anatomy. Commercially available SD-OCT devices include: the Cirrus OCT made by Carl Zeiss Meditech, the Spectralis OCT made by Heidelberg Engineering, 3D-OCT 1000 (Topcon), Bioptigen SD OCT (Bioptogen) and the RT-Vue (Optovue).

Swept Source OCT

In swept source (or optical frequency domain) OCT scanning, the light source is rapidly swept in wavelength and the spectral interference pattern is detected on a single or small number of receivers as a function of time. The spectral interference patterns obtained as a function of time then undergo a reverse Fourier transform to generate an A-scan image. Higher scanning speeds allow for denser sampling and better registration. The swept source OCT also has less sensitivity roll-off with depth, allowing better visualization of structures deep to the retina. At present, swept source OCT is not widely available commercially with the DRI-OCT 1 (Topcon) being the only commercially available device.

Scanning Principles

1.2 Basic Scan Patterns and OCT Output

Each commercially available OCT device has unique scan patterns that are programmed into the machine. There is considerable overlap between devices, however, with several general scan patterns available across all devices. The scan patterns for the major commercially available machines are summarized in Table 1.2.1. The two most commonly used scans in evaluating retinal disease are:

▸ Macular cube scan
▸ Line scan(s)

Depending on the particular machine, scan patterns may be programmable with respect to functions such as pixel density, B-scan density, speed, ability to oversample, and length of scanned image.

Macular Cube Scan

Cube scans are 'volume' or '3D' scans analogous to computed tomography or magnetic resonance scans that acquire volumetric cubes of data. SD-OCT machines acquire a rapid series of line scans (B-scans), generally in a 6 mm × 6 mm square area centered on the fovea. The scans are generally at relatively lower resolution, in order to minimize the time of scanning. As a result, when examining individual line scans from a cube scan, some detail is lost. As a default the cube scan is centered at the fovea, but other areas of interest can be captured by manually centering the scan elsewhere in the retina. Optic nerve topographic scans are cube scans centered on the nerve.

In the Zeiss Cirrus SD-OCT, there are two macular cube scans available, with no ability to customize. Both scans capture a 6 mm × 6 mm area centered at the macula. There is a faster 200 × 200 cube (200 B-scans each comprised of 200 A-scans) or the slightly slower 512 × 128 cube (128 B-scans each comprised of 512 A-scans) that has higher quality horizontal scans. The 'volume scan' on the Heidelberg Spectralis uses a similar raster scanning protocol with a 'fast' 25 B-scans each consisting of 512 sample points or A-scans, or with a 'dense' 1024 × 49 default scanning protocol. The Topcon 3D OCT uses a 256 × 256 or a 512 × 128 scanning protocol. The RT-Vue '3D macular scan' consists of a 4 mm × 4 mm macular cube scan with 101 B-scans consisting of 512 A-scans each, and the MM5 protocol uses a mix of vertical and horizontal B-scans to create a grid-like (not true raster) scanning pattern.

▸ **Raster Scans**: raster scanning is one method used to obtain cube scans of the macula. This involves a systematic pattern of image capture over a rectangular area using closely spaced parallel lines. It leads to a uniform sampling density over the entire area being scanned with the OCT.

▸ **Radial Scans**: these consist of six to 12 high resolution line scans taken at radial orientations, all passing through the fovea. The RT-Vue's MM6 is a radial line scanning pattern with 12 lines radially oriented to the fovea, each 6 mm long. The macular radial scanning pattern of the Spectralis and the 6-line radial scan of the Topcon 3D OCT 100 are similar. A disadvantage of the radial line scans is that the machine interpolates between the scans when generating macular thickness maps. This is reasonable for the fovea where the lines are close to each other, but can miss lesions further out in the macula where the lines are spaced further apart.

4

Basic Scan Patterns and OCT Output

	Zeiss Cirrus	Heidelberg Spectralis	RT-Vue	Topcon 3-D	Canon HS-100	Nidek OCT RS-3000	Bioptogen SD-OCT
3D scans	Macular cube	Volume scan	3D macular MM5	Fast map Box scan	Macula 3D Multi-cross	Macula map	Rectangular volume Mixed volume
Line scans	5-line raster scan 1-line raster scan	7-line raster scan	Line scan HD Line Cross-line HD cross-Line	5- and 9- line raster Line scan Oversampled line scan	Cross	Macula multi Macula line	Linear scan
Radial scans	None	No presets, can be selected	Radial slicer MM6	12-line radial		Macula radial	Radial volume
Mesh scan	None		MM5			Macula multi	

Table 1.2.1 Scan patterns in commonly used OCT devices

▶ **Mesh Scans**: Some machines include a mesh scanning pattern that acquire vertical and horizontal B-scans over the area of interest. The MM5 protocol of the RT-Vue uses a less dense outer and a more dense inner grid. The outer grid has horizontal and vertical B-scans 0.5 mm apart and the inner grid has horizontal and vertical B-scans each 0.1 mm apart.

Line, Cross-Line and Raster Scans

SD-OCT line scans are a single B-scan composed of generally a higher number of A-scans than the cube scans. This higher sampling density allows higher resolution scans of the retinal tissue to be acquired. In addition, oversampling can be performed to increase signal-noise ratio (Fig. 1.2.1). The Cirrus 5-line raster consists of five horizontal 6 mm lines each scanned four times and averaged. The five lines in the raster can be collapsed to obtain a single line scan that consists of 20 averaged B-scans. The 'cross-line' scan of the RT-Vue consists of a horizontal and vertical line scan while the 7-line raster of the Heidelberg also spans a 6 mm × 6 mm area of the macula. Heidelberg can be programmed to oversample a line scan up to 100 times at each point.

Enhanced Depth Imaging

Enhanced depth imaging (EDI) protocols, now available in all major commercial OCT devices, use a combination of image averaging and of moving the zero delay line of the SD-OCT closer to the choroid, to obtain higher resolution images of the choroid. EDI is invaluable in diseases that involve the choroid where somewhat higher choroidal resolution is needed, as well as diseases with choroidal thickening where the sclerochoroidal border may not be visible on standard scanning protocols

Macular Maps

Macular maps are derived directly from either the cube scan data or radial scans, depending on the machine. They come in two forms:
▶ numeric displays showing the average retinal thickness in the zone of interest
▶ color-coded displays illustrating the difference between the examination and age-matched normative data base (Fig. 1.2.2).

C-Scans (*En Face* Images), OCT Fundus Image (Rendered Fundus Image, Summed Voxel Projection [SVP])

This image looks like a red-free image of the retina and is obtained by summation of data from all the B-scans. It is currently available in all SD-OCT machines except Heidelberg (Fig. 1.2.3).

Topographical maps

Retinal thickness data obtained from segmented 3D datasets are used to form a 2D topographical data set that can be displayed in false color (color-coded) displays, or as an overlay on the OCT rendered fundus image to obtain a quick topographic picture of the macula, internal limiting membrane or retinal pigment epithelium layer (Fig. 1.2.4).

6

Segmented 3D datasets over the optic nerve can be used to generate nerve fiber layer thickness measurements that can then be compared to age matched controls and displayed in a color-coded pattern (Fig. 1.2.5).

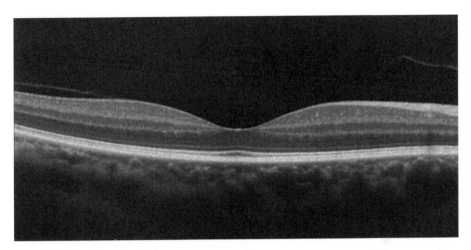

Figure 1.2.1 Line scan through the macula.

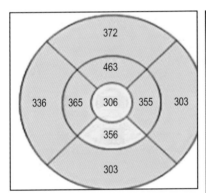

Figure 1.2.2 Macular map showing retinal thickness.

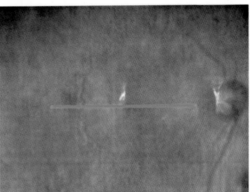

Figure 1.2.3 *En face* image or a summed voxel projection.

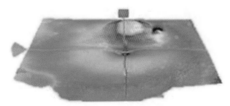

Figure 1.2.4 Topographical map.

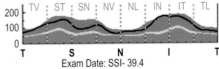

Figure 1.2.5 Retinal nerve fiber layer analysis.

2.1 OCT Interpretation

OCT interpretation can be both qualitative and quantitative. At present, in order to fully evaluate an OCT image, both are important.

Qualitative Interpretation

In qualitative interpretation, the clinician reviews individual line scans (B-scans) imaging the areas of interest in the retina and makes qualitative assessment of the presence or absence of pathology based on a knowledge of normal anatomy. B-scans can be rendered in a color-coded image or in a gray-scale image representing the reflectivity of the various layers. By comparing line scans performed over time, the course of the underlying disease and its response to treatment can be assessed.

When performing qualitative interpretation, it is important to be aware of the following issues:

▶ **Registration**: future line scans must be 'registered' to past scans. In other words, the examiner must be certain that the precise anatomic area of interest is scanned similarly in future tests. All SD-OCT machines have the capability of registering future line scans to past scans.

▶ **Sampling error**: if only one or several line scans are examined, the true pathology may be missed. It is important when doing qualitative interpretation that multiple line scans through the macula are examined.

▶ **Subjective evaluation**: by its nature, the lack of accurate quantitative numbers mean that line scan interpretation will be individualized. In addition, it is hard to gauge the effects of pathology that is improving in one area of the macula but getting worse in another.

Zones of line scans can be qualitatively described as hyper-reflective or hyporeflective, and demonstrate 'shadowing' or 'reverse shadowing.' **Hyper-reflective** areas reflect more light than normal for a given region. On the grey-scale image, they appear whiter than the surrounding areas. Examples include epiretinal membranes and hard exudates. **Hypore-flective** areas reflect less light than the surrounding areas. Areas with a higher fluid content, e.g. intraretinal cysts, are usually hyporeflective. **Shadowing** occurs when there is increased absorption of light compared to the surrounding tissue. This causes optical shadowing and decreased visualization of the outer tissues. Vitreous debris, larger retinal vessels, hard exudates and highly pigmented areas cause shadowing. **Reverse shadowing** occurs when there is loss/atrophy of pigmented tissue that allows excessive light to be transmitted through to the outer layers. The retinal pigment epithelium (RPE) is a major source of light absorption on OCT scanning, so atrophy of the RPE can cause reverse shadowing.

Quantitative Interpretation

Quantitative interpretation of OCT scans relies on the ability of the OCT software to distinguish the inner and outer margins of the retina or sub-layers (e.g. nerve fiber layer), referred to as segmentation, and accurately calculate retinal thickness and/or volume. Retinal thickness can then be compared to age-matched controls for assessment of normalcy, and monitored over time to judge the progression or regression of disease. Newer generation OCT software features the ability to register subsequent OCT scans so that measurements of retinal thickness are compared over the same area of the macula every time. These are usually presented as Early Treatment of Diabetic Retinopathy Study grids or color-coded maps of retinal thickness.

When comparing quantitative OCT scans, it is important to compare scans obtained on the same machine, since different OCT machines draw the outer retinal boundary at different levels (inner segment–outer segment [IS-OS] photoreceptor junction, OS tips, RPE) and therefore may obtain different retinal thickness measurements on the same patient at the same visit.

The major drawback to quantitative assessment is that even in modern SD-OCT machines, quantitative scans are prone to artifacts. For example, the machine software may inaccurately identify the inner or outer retinal boundaries and the thickness measurement is therefore inaccurate. This is called software breakdown. Artifacts can induce errors in measurement making quantitative data inaccurate.

3.1 Artifacts on OCT

Artifacts can occur during image acquisition or analysis due to software, patient or operator factors. Artifacts may affect the qualitative or quantitative interpretation of images and are therefore important to identify.

▸ **Mirror artifact** (Fig 3.1.1): this artifact is unique to SD-OCT. It occurs when the area of interest to be imaged crosses the zero delay line and results in an inverted image. In practical terms, this happens when the OCT machine is pushed too close to the eye, or when the eye has pathology (e.g. retinoschisis or high myopia) in which a large axial range has to be imaged. The resulting image is inverted, partly inverted or may possibly have poor resolution.

▸ **Vignetting** (Fig. 3.1.2): this occurs when a part of the OCT beam is blocked by the iris and is characterized by a loss of signal over one side of the image.

▸ **Misalignment** (Fig. 3.1.3): this occurs when the fovea is not properly aligned during a volumetric scan. Typically it is due to the patient exhibiting poor or eccentic fixation or poor attention. When misalignment occurs, the normal foveal depression will not appear aligned with the center of the ETDRS map.

▸ **Software breakdown** (Fig. 3.1.4): software breakdown results from misidentification of the inner or outer retinal boundaries causing incorrectly drawn OCT segmentation lines, resulting in inaccurate mapping and quantitative measurements in a volumetric scan. These errors are more common in TD-OCT than in SD-OCT.

Inner line breakdown typically happens in vitreomacular surface disorders such as vitreomacular traction or epiretinal membrane formation, while outer line breakdown happens in conditions involving the outer retina/retinal pigment epithelium such as central serous chorioretinopathy (CSCR), age-related macular dystrophy, cystoid macular edema and retinal atrophy. In pathologies such as CSCR where retinal thickness maps drive therapeutic decisions, these errors may be critically important.

▸ **Blink artifact** (Fig. 3.1.5): blink artifacts result in partial loss of data due to the momentary blockage of OCT image acquisition during the blink. Blink artifacts are easily recognized as black horizontal bars across the OCT image and macular map. Lubrication with artificial tears and/or protocols using shorter acquisition times may help to avoid these.

▸ **Motion artifact** (Fig. 3.1.5): this occurs when there is movement of the eye during OCT scanning leading to distortion or double scanning of the same area. It is seen as a sharp change in contour on the B-scan and as misalignment of blood vessels and blurring on the en face scans. Motion artifacts can occur because of poor fixation, tracking of the light source, heartbeat, respiration, drifts or saccades. It can cause errors especially in quantitative measurements. Mechanical tracking or software innovations can minimize motion artifact.

▸ **Out of range error** (Fig. 3.1.6): this error occurs because the B-scan is vertically shifted out of the scanning range (e.g. by the scanner being too close or too far away from the eye of the subject), causing a section of the OCT scan to be cut off.

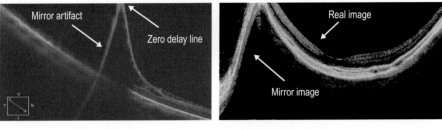

Figure 3.1.1 Mirror artifact occurring in a case of retinoschisis (above) and a high myopic eye with a long axial length. The inverted image can be seen adjacent to the regular image.

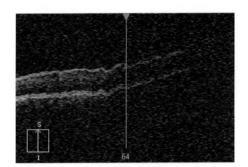

Figure 3.1.2 Vignetting is seen with loss of signal over the right side of the image.

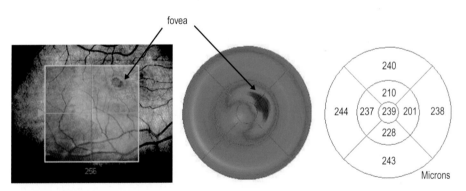

Figure 3.1.3 Misalignment error. Note that the fovea is not centered on the Early Treatment of Diabetic Retinopathy Study grid. On the macular thickness map, the thinnest point of the macula is decentered off the center of the map.

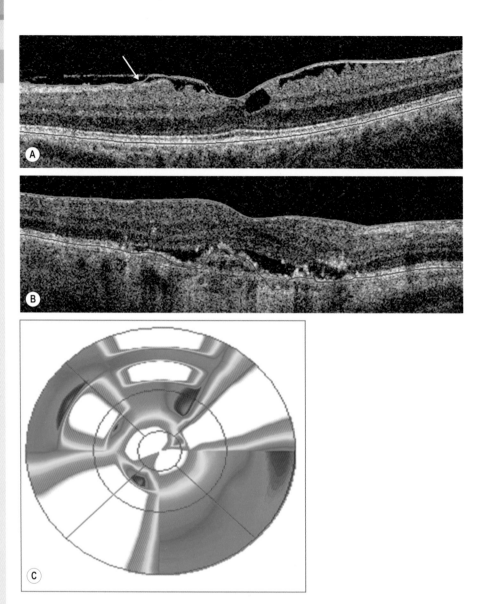

Figure 3.1.4 Software breakdown. Note the inaccuracy of tracing of the (A) inner retinal line (green) in a patient with epiretinal membrane, and (B) of the outer retinal/retinal pigment epithelium line (blue). (C) Software breakdown should be suspected when the macular thickness map shows a bowtie configuration or isolated islands of thinning and thickening.

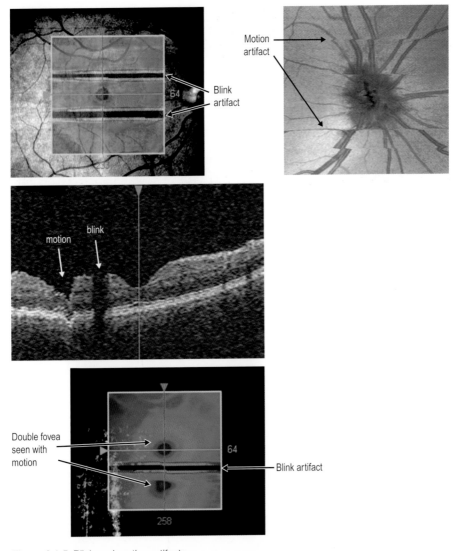

Figure 3.1.5 Blink and motion artifacts.

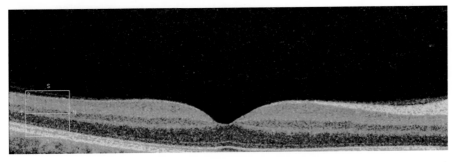

Figure 3.1.6 Out of range error. Notice that the outer retina/choroidal image is cut off because of improper positioning of the machine during image acquisition.

4.1 Normal Retinal Anatomy and Basic Pathologic Appearances

Normal Retinal Anatomy

Commercially available SD-OCT scanners have an axial resolution of between 4 μm and 7 μm and a transverse resolution of approximately 15 μm. This high resolution allows for exquisite viewing of the retinal detail. Due to the limited penetration of light beyond the pigmented RPE and the drop-off of the OCT signal with depth, the image at the level of the choroid has lower resolution. The layers of the normal retina are labeled in Figure 4.1.1.

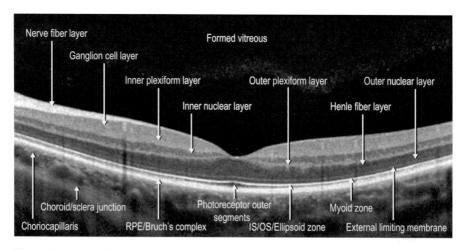

Figure 4.1.1 Normal retinal anatomy.

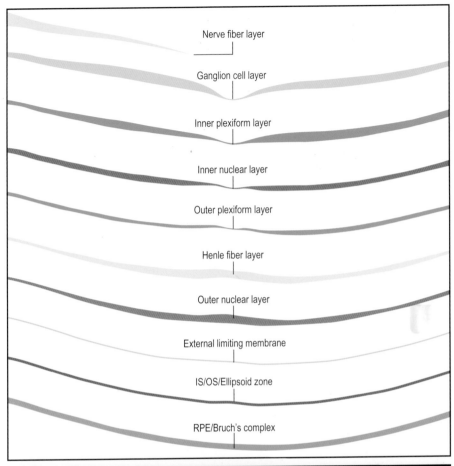

Nerve fiber layer

Ganglion cell layer

Inner plexiform layer

Inner nuclear layer

Outer plexiform layer

Henle fiber layer

Outer nuclear layer

External limiting membrane

IS/OS/Ellipsoid zone

RPE/Bruch's complex

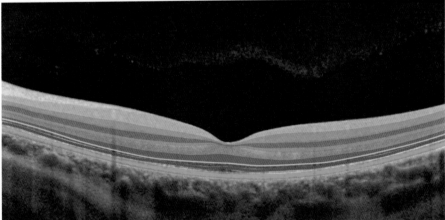

Figure 4.1.1 *Continued.*

Additional Vitreous Features

Some additional vitreous features are demonstrated in a normal OCT scan in Figure 4.1.2:

▸ Posterior cortical vitreous (posterior hyaloid)
▸ Retro-hyaloidal space

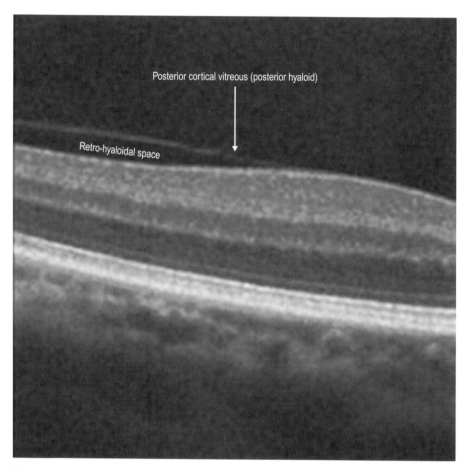

Figure 4.1.2 Vitreous features in a normal eye with partial, shallow vitreous separation.

Cystic Changes in Outer Retina

Discrete hyporeflective spaces are noticed primarily in the outer retina, but usually span multiple layers (Fig. 4.1.3).

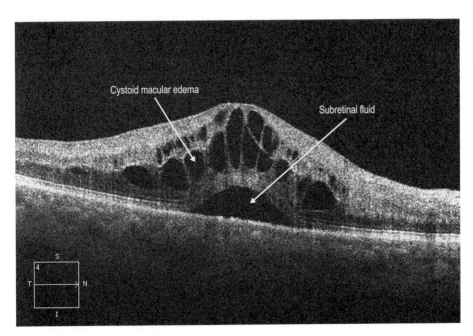

Figure 4.1.3 Cystoid changes in retina.

The differential diagnosis includes:
- Diabetic macular edema
- Branch retinal vein occlusion
- Central retinal vein occlusion
- Retinal telangiectasias (e.g. Coat's disease, macular telangiectasia)
- Retinitis pigmentosa
- Uveitis/retinal vasculitis
- Post surgery
- Nicotinic acid maculopathy
- Vitreomacular disorders (vitreomacular traction, epiretinal membrane)
- Chronic subretinal fluid (e.g. retinal detachment, choroidal neovasclar membrane, central serous chorioretinopathy)
- Idiopathic.

Subretinal Fluid

Clear hyporeflective space seen between the neurosensory retina and the RPE (Fig. 4.1.4).

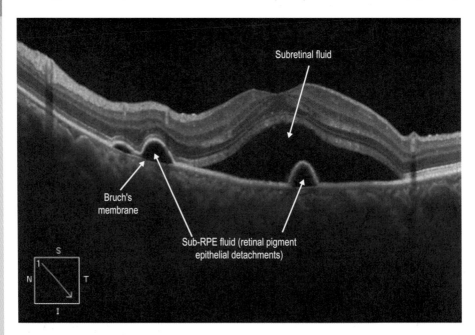

Figure 4.1.4 Clear subretinal fluid.

The differential diagnosis includes:
▸ Central serous chorioretinopathy
▸ Choroidal neovascular membranes (secondary to e.g. age-related macular degeneration, myopia)
▸ Serous retinal detachments (secondary to tumors, inflammation, trauma)
▸ Rhegmatogenous retinal detachment
▸ Tractional retinal detachment.

TURBID SUBRETINAL FLUID

Subretinal fluid may be turbid or have a higher reflectivity than the vitreous in conditions where there is fibrin deposition in the subretinal space (Fig. 4.1.5).

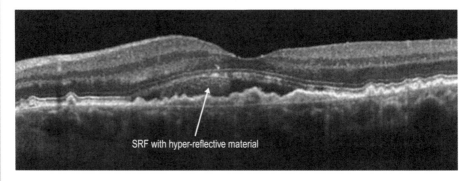

Figure 4.1.5 Turbid subretinal fluid (SRF).

The differential diagnosis includes

- Chronic central serous chorioretinopathy
- Chronic choroidal neovascular membrane
- Sympathetic ophthalmia
- Vogt–Koyanagi–Harada syndrome
- Inflammatory serous retinal detachments.

Retinal Pigment Epithelial Detachment

This is noted as a dome-shaped separation of the RPE from the underlying Bruch's membrane. The ensuing space between the RPE and the Bruch's membrane is hyporeflective (Fig. 4.1.6).

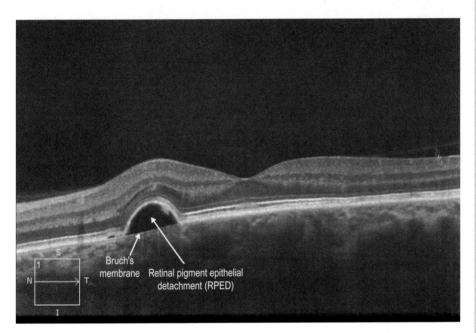

Figure 4.1.6 Retinal pigment epithelial detachment.

The differential diagnosis includes:

- Age-related macular degeneration
- Central serous chorioretinopathy
- Choroidal neovascularization (e.g myopic degeneration, presumed ocular histoplasmosis, angioid streaks)
- Idiopathic.

RPE Atrophy

Atrophy of the pigmented RPE causes decreased absorption of light. The OCT signal is therefore able to penetrate more deeply, which exaggerates the typical signal pattern so that there is a 'reverse' shadowing effect (Fig. 4.1.7, area between the smaller arrows)

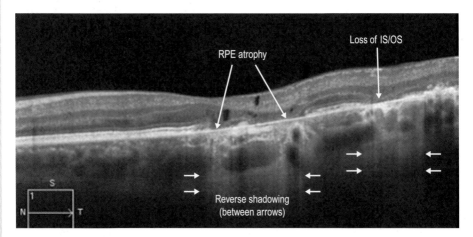

Figure 4.1.7 RPE atrophy and loss of photoreceptors with mild cystic change in the retina.

The differential diagnosis includes:
▸ Geographic atrophy secondary to age-related macular degeneration
▸ Advanced chorioretinal scarring secondary to retinal degenerations and macular dytrophies (e.g. retinitis pigmentosa, Stargardt's disease, cone dystrophy)
▸ Chorioretinal atrophy secondary to inflammatory disorders (e.g. ocular histoplasmosis, multifocal choroiditis)
▸ Severe myopic degeneration
▸ Angioid streaks.

Focal Loss of External Limiting Membrane (ELM) and Inner Segment–Outer Segment (IS–OS) Photoreceptor Junction

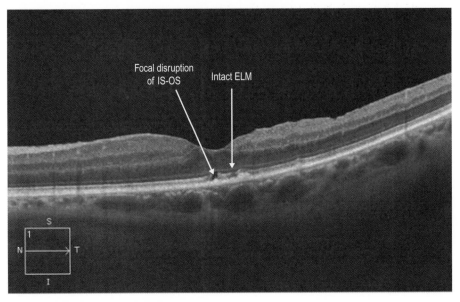

Figure 4.1.8 Focal loss of IS–OS/ellipsoid layer.

OCT scanning reveals a disruption in the ELM line and in the IS–OS junction (Fig. 4.1.8). This is associated with a number of severe outer retinal conditions such as cone dystrophy and solar retinopathy as well as inner retinal disorders when they advance to involving the outer retinal layers. Loss of the IS–OS junction/ellipsoid layer as well as ELM has been associated with reduction in visual acuity and a worse prognosis for visual recovery in a number of ocular disorders.

Normal Retinal Anatomy and Basic Pathologic Appearances

Vitreous Opacities

Posterior vitreous opacities are seen as hyper-reflective specks in the vitreous space (Fig. 4.1.9).

The differential diagnosis includes:

▸ Vitritis
▸ Asteroid hyalosis
▸ Syneresis scintillans
▸ Operculum (e.g. related to a macular hole)
▸ Fungal hyphae.

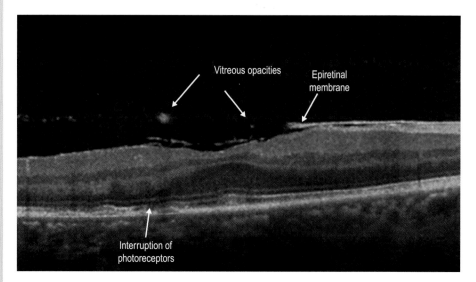

Figure 4.1.9 Vitreous opacities.

PART 2: Optic Nerve Disorders

5.1 | Basic Optic Nerve Scan Patterns and Output

The commercially available SD-OCT machines have two basic scan patterns used to evaluate the optic nerve:

▸ **Volume scans**: these are analogous to macular cube scans in which a volumetric set of data is acquired, centered at the optic nerve head. These may be square or rectangular cubes of data, or cylindrical cubes acquired by circumferential scanning around the optic nerve. The Cirrus HD-OCT scanning protocol acquires a 6 mm × 6 mm cube of data at the optic nerve head using a series of rapid B-scans (200 × 200). Software processing within the SD-OCT machine then identifies the center of the optic disc and creates a 3.46 mm circle centered on this location for registration purposes. The data set is then used to measure retinal nerve fiber layer thickness. The Heidelberg Spectralis volumetric scanning protocols acquire a set of three sequential circular scans, each with 256 axial scans, centered at the optic nerve head. This yields a cylindrical volume with a diameter of 3.4 mm through and around the optic nerve head.

Occasionally, the concentric circular scanning protocol can be accompanied by the addition of radial line scans that allow for better registration of the concentric scans. The RTVue's optic nerve head scan pattern consists of a grid pattern with circular and radial scans that acquires a 4 mm × 4 mm volume around the optic nerve. Some machines also have the ability to acquire ganglion cell complex scans as part of the glaucoma imaging protocol, that look at cubes of data centered on the macula.

▸ **Line Scans**: a single or a series of high-resolution B-scans can be obtained through the optic nerve head similar to the line scans obtained in the macula, to allow for higher resolution visualization of structure and pathology at the optic nerve head. Line scans are most frequently used in the qualitative interpretation of data and the identification of anatomic anomalies.

Volume scans obtained through the optic nerve head are processed to delineate the optic disc margin and optic disc surface contour and segmented to obtain the retinal nerve fiber layer (NFL) boundaries. Since most OCT measurements of the optic nerve head are highly sensitive to scan position, all commercially available OCT devices have motion correction software. The information obtained from the optic nerve volumetric scans is processed to obtain the following details.

RNFL thickness is calculated by the OCT devices as the distance between the internal limiting membrane and the outer aspect of the NFL (Fig. 5.1.1). Because the RNFL varies with distance from the center of the optic nerve, most machines use a circle of a pre-defined diameter (usually between 3.4–3.46 mm) around the center of the optic nerve as the reference point at which to calculate RNFL thickness. One of the reasons that measurement of the RNFL between machines is not comparable is that different machines use circles of different diameters around the center of the optic nerve head.

RNFL thickness is then compared to age, ethnicity and disk size-matched normative databases. The results are displayed in various forms including a false color scale where green represents normal, yellow represents a 'borderline' RNFL thickness (less than a 5% probability of being normal), and red represents an abnormal RNFL thickness with less than a 1% probability of being normal. Results from the two eyes are also compared and any discrepancy between the two is highlighted. The RNFL thickness may be displayed as an average for the overall map, for quadrants, sectors, hemispheres or clock hours.

One of the most useful RNFL displays in clinical practice is the sinusoidal signal profile wave corresponding to the RNFL thickness profile 360° around the optic nerve, starting from the temporal region and proceeding through the superior, inferior, nasal and back to the temporal region (TSINT). This normally presents a 'double hump' pattern corresponding to the superior and inferior quadrants, where the RNFL is thickest. The inferior and superior quadrant RNFL thickness has been demonstrated to be the most useful in glaucoma diagnosis.

Optic Nerve Morphology

The software in various SD-OCT machines also calculates and displays areas for the optic disc, cup and rim, volumes for optic nerve head, cup and rim, cup-to-disc ratios and cup-to-disc horizontal and vertical ratios (Fig. 5.1.2).

Basic Optic Nerve Scan Patterns and Output

The ganglion cell complex consists of three inner retinal layers: the NFL (formed by axons of the ganglion cells), the ganglion cell layer (cell body of the ganglion cells) and the inner plexiform layer (dendrites of the ganglion cells). The GCC scan is a series of B-scans centered on the macula and quantifies the thickness in all of these three layers. After image processing, GCC thickness is calculated as the distance between the internal limiting membrane and the outer boundary of the inner plexiform layer. The software presents the results as a color-coded 'map', which compares the examined eye with a normative data-base and indicates deviations from the normal values (Figs 5.1.2 and 5.1.3). The GCC scan must be precisely centered at the fovea to have its results compared with a normative database, or to permit progression analysis.

The GCC thickness analysis may be displayed as an average overall thickness, averages in the superior and inferior hemiretina, superior–inferior difference in GCC thickness, the global loss volume (integration of all negative deviation values normalized by the overall map area), and the focal loss volume (integration of negative deviation values in the areas of significant focal loss).

FIGURE LEGENDS

Figure 5.1.1 SD-OCT scan in the macular area with the RNFL highlighted in red.
The peripapillary RNFL thickness is calculated according to the distance between the internal limiting membrane and the outer aspect of the RNFL.

Figure 5.1.2 Composite figure showing the right and left optic disc photographs (top) and OCT printout (bottom) of a normal individual. The optic disc area is 1.53 mm^2 and 1.58 mm^2 for the right and left optic disc, respectively. For this individual all retinal nerve fiber layer and ganglion cell complex parameters are colored green, indicating the patient is likely normal. The right bottom TSINT graph shows the results from both eyes plotted together. Any statistically significant asymmetry between the two eyes is shown in color between the two lines on the plots.

Figure 5.1.3 Composite figure showing the right and left optic disc photographs (top) and OCT printout (bottom) of a patient with glaucoma. Both optic discs show an increase in the cup-to-disc ratio with loss of neuroretinal rim tissue on the inferior aspect of the optic disc. The optic nerve head map shows substantial retinal nerve fiber layer thinning in the inferotemporal sector in both eyes, with a corresponding thinning of the ganglion cell complex in the inferior macula.

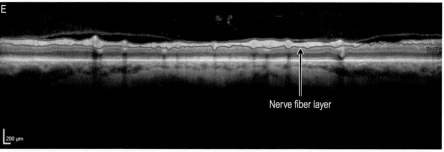

Figure 5.1.1

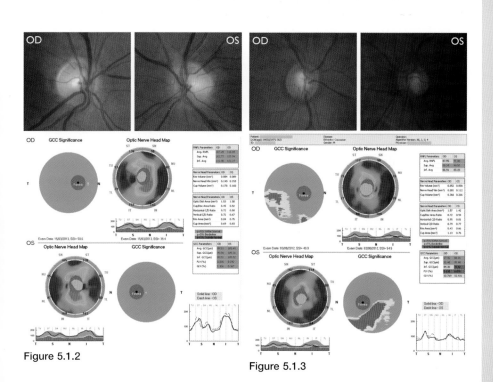

Figure 5.1.2

Figure 5.1.3

6.1 Glaucoma

Introduction: Glaucoma is a progressive optic neuropathy characterized by loss of retinal ganglion cells with resulting progressive visual field loss. It is the leading cause of irreversible blindness worldwide.

Retinal ganglion cell bodies are located in the ganglion cell layer of the inner retina. Their axons constitute the RNFL. The axons extend in an arcuate pattern to converge at the optic nerve head (ONH). Glaucoma is a heterogeneous condition, with variable pathophysiological mechanisms culminating in retinal ganglion cell loss and optic atrophy. The most prevalent type is primary open angle glaucoma. Mechanical factors at the level of the optic nerve head, genetic susceptibility and oxidative stress are hypothesized to be involved.

Clinical Features: The hallmark of glaucomatous optic neuropathy is a progressive loss of RNFL tissue eventually culminating in visual field loss, with associated changes in the ONH (Fig. 6.1.1). This may be associated with elevated intraocular pressure. The RNFL loss can be noted qualitatively on careful clinical examination, and is best appreciated with red-free illumination of the fundus. Slit-lamp biomicroscopy with a handheld lens is the best method of optic disc examination, since it provides good stereopsis and magnification. Optic disc stereo photographs are complementary and may identify findings missed on slit-lamp examination. Progressive changes in the ONH follow the RNFL loss, including focal or diffuse loss of neuroretinal rim tissue and enlargement of the cup.

OCT Features: OCT has become a valuable tool in the initial diagnosis of glaucoma and subsequent monitoring of disease progression over time. OCT scans represent non-invasive, reproducible measurements of the structural changes that occur in glaucoma. OCT permits quantitative documentation and analysis of the areas most affected by glaucoma: the ONH, the peripapillary retina, and the macular retina.

The key anatomical features assessed on the ONH scan are:
▸ RNFL thickness
▸ optic disc rim
▸ optic disc cup (Fig. 6.1.1C,D,E)

Additionally, glaucomatous damage to the ganglion cells of the macula and the resultant overall **macular retinal thinning** can be assessed with GCC mapping. The diagnosis of glaucoma is improved by the analysis of GCC compared to measurement of full retinal thickness.

Most commercially available OCT machines have software permitting comparison of change over time.

Ancillary Testing: Visual field testing estimates the functional damage in glaucomatous eyes. However, it has been shown that up to 50% of the RNFL may be lost prior to any change in the visual field. Moreover, visual field testing is dependent on patient cooperation and often exhibits large variation between visits. Detection of visual field changes often requires several repetitions of the test, which may delay the diagnosis (Fig. 6.1.1B).

Treatment: Treatment strategy is directed toward improving the parameters that cause further damage to the nerve fiber layer. Primarily this involves lowering intraocular pressures. Neuroprotection is also a large area of research in glaucoma.

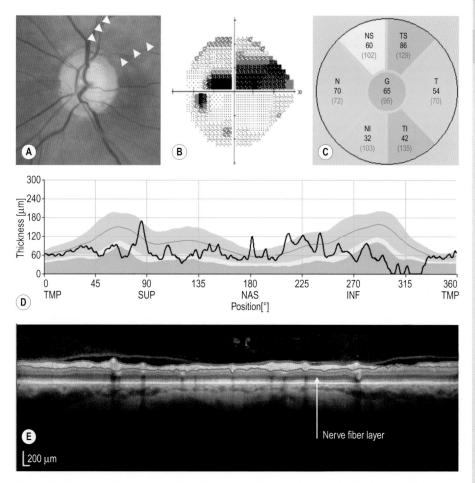

Figure 6.1.1 Composite figure showing (A) the left optic disc photograph, (B) the visual field, (C) the six sectors OCT map, (D) the TSINT map, and (E) the OCT scan with the RNFL automated segmentation of a patient with moderate glaucoma (visual field mean deviation −6.4 dB). The optic disc (A) shows an inferotemporal focal absence of neuroretinal rim tissue (notch) and superotemporal focal thinning of the neuroretinal rim tissue (notching) with the corresponding RNFL defect (between arrowheads). The visual field (B) shows a defect in the superior hemifield threatening fixation. The OCT (C, D and E) shows markedly RNFL thinning of the superotemporal and inferotemporal sectors with 'outside normal limits' classification for both and 'borderline' classification in the superonasal sector. The OCT scan shows pronounced RNFL thinning in the inferotemporal sector, noticed in the segmented RNFL (arrow in E). *(Courtesy of Dr Marcelo Nicolela, Dalhousie University.)*

6.2 | Optic Neuropathies and Papilledema

The diagnosis of optic neuropathy is typically made on clinical basis. The history and pattern of onset of an optic neuropathy often points to the diagnosis and etiology, with a rapid onset typical of demyelinating, inflammatory, ischemic and traumatic causes, while a gradual onset is more suggestive of compressive, toxic/nutritional and some hereditary causes.

Clinical features characteristic of optic neuropathies include afferent pupillary defect, vision loss of varying degrees, dyschromatopsia and visual field defects. Ancillary testing in optic neuropathies includes visual field testing, and the pattern of the visual field defect is often characteristic of the underlying disease. Neuroimaging is also often critical to the diagnosis of optic neuropathies. OCT is emerging as an increasingly important ancillary test in the diagnosis and follow-up of disorders of the optic nerve. OCT patterns vary depending on the clinical findings of the optic neuropathy as well as its stage. Since many optic neuropathies manifest as disc edema and/or optic nerve head atrophy, the characteristic OCT findings in these are summarized below.

OPTIC NEURITIS

Optic neuritis or inflammation of the optic nerve is the most common cause of optic neuropathy in young adults. Optic neuritis can be idiopathic or associated with demyelinating lesions (e.g. multiple sclerosis), infectious and para-infectious conditions, inflammatory and post-vaccination conditions and autoimmune diseases. OCT B-scans through the optic nerve head can document **disc edema** in acute optic neuritis. Optic nerve head and retinal nerve fiber layer thickening analysis can reflect changes related to optic disc edema, as well as progressive changes related to long-term **axonal loss** and **optic atrophy** (Fig. 6.2.1).

DISC EDEMA/PAPILLEDEMA

Optic nerve head swelling or disc edema occurs in many pathologic conditions of the optic nerve. It is thought to represent a stasis in axoplasmic flow through the retinal nerve fiber layer due to biochemical and structural reasons and manifests itself by swelling and thickening of the retinal nerve fiber layer. Papilledema is edema of the optic nerve due to elevated intracranial pressure (ICP). OCT features include **increased total retinal thickness** and **retinal nerve fiber layer (RNFL) thickness** on the optic nerve volumetric scan. The total retinal thickness is more sensitive than the RNFL thickness both in early cases of papilledema where RNFL thickness may miss some cases, as well as in cases of severe edema where software breakdown on retinal segmentation may give inaccurate values of RNFL thickness (Fig. 6.2.2). Recent studies suggest that increased thickening of the peripapillary RNFL is associated with increased ICP in newly diagnosed patients with papilledema. In patients with long-term severe papilledema, SD-OCT appears to be of limited value in predicting increased ICP. Interestingly, it has been shown on B-scans through the optic nerve head that some patients with papilledema may exhibit **inward angulation** of the peripapillary RPE/Bruch's membrane (BM) layer at the neural canal opening, which does not occur in other causes of disc edema.

OPTIC ATROPHY

This is the final common pathway for many optic nerve disorders. Nerve fiber layer scans show **thinning** of the RNFL. OCT measurements of peripapillary RNFL thickness and of macular retinal ganglion cell thickness can also be affected, starting in early stages of the disease (Fig. 6.2.3).

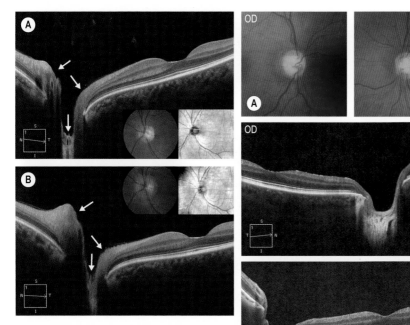

Figure 6.2.1 (A) Line scan through the optic nerve of a patient with multiple sclerosis and no optic neuritis with a relatively normal optic nerve and (B) the same patient at the time of optic neuritis showing significant disc edema. Arrows correspond to similar locations, for comparison.

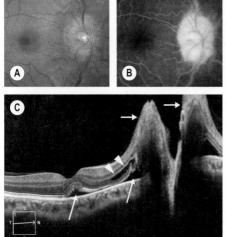

Figure 6.2.2 (A) Photograph of papilledema in the setting of increased ICP. (B) Fluorescein angiography shows significant late leakage from the optic nerve head. (C) OCT line scan shows profound optic disc thickening (short arrows), subretinal fluid (long arrows), and cystoid macular edema (arrowheads).

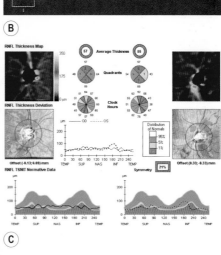

Figure 6.2.3 (A) Color fundus photographs and a (B) B-scan through the optic nerve head of a patient with optic atrophy. OCT B-scans through the optic nerve head show enlarged cupping in both eyes due to retinal ganglion cell's axonal loss, and optic nerve head and (C) RNFL analysis shows abnormally reduced RNFL thickness in both eyes.

6.3 | Congenital Optic Nerve Head Abnormalities

Several structural abnormalities of the optic nerve have been described on OCT scanning. All occur rarely.

OPTIC DISC COLOBOMA

Optic disc colobomas are uncommon congenital defects that develop as a result of defective closure of the fetal fissure (Fig. 6.3.1). Colobomas can be associated with peripapillary retinal detachments or schisis. In posterior segment colobomas, histological and OCT studies show that a tissue called the **intercalary membrane** overlies the area affected by the defect. OCT allows a qualitative assessment of the vitreous in eyes with optic disc colobomas, documenting the degree of **vitreous condensation** and adhesion in the area of the optic disc, especially with the three-dimensional reconstruction. OCT can potentially reveal **retinal breaks** on the optic disc margin. **Retinal detachments** and **schisis** associated with the optic disc colobomas can also be visualized on OCT scanning.

OPTIC DISC PIT

Optic disc pit is a rare congenital anomaly of the optic nerve head (Fig. 6.3.2). Associated maculopathy has been reported to eventually develop in over 90% of affected eyes. OCT line scans through the affected regions show both **subretinal fluid** and **schisis** of the outer retinal layers, extending from the temporal margin of the disc to the nasal aspect of the fovea, and overlying a central neurosensory retinal detachment. **Lamellar macular holes** or even **full-thickness macular holes** can develop.

OPTIC NERVE HEAD DRUSEN

ONH drusen are not an unusual congenital and developmental abnormalities (Fig. 6.3.3). Drusen exhibit shadowing on the OCT B-scan. Optical coherence tomography is valuable in the diagnosis of ONH drusen, and in the differential diagnosis with ONH edema. The **retinal nerve fiber layer (RNFL) thickness and the peripapillary total retinal thickness** are significantly greater in eyes with ONH edema than in eyes with ONH drusen. A recent study suggests that EDI may be more efficient than regular OCT scanning in detecting ONH drusen.

MEGALOPAPILLA

Megalopapilla is a congenital malformation characterized by an abnormally large optic disc, with no pathological significance (Fig. 6.3.4). The RNFL thickness is **normal** in megalopapilla, which is an essential feature in the differential diagnosis with glaucomatous optic neuropathy. Normative data from normal eyes indicate that the RNFL is thicker in superior and inferior fundus quadrants, while it is thinner in nasal and temporal quadrants. The same features are observed in eyes with megalopapilla.

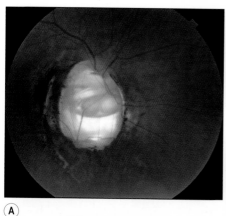

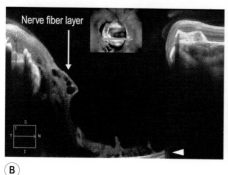

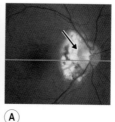

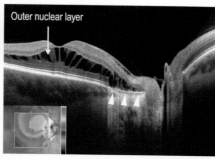

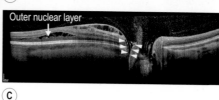

Figure 6.3.1 Color photograph of an optic disc coloboma of the right eye. There is minimal retinal involvement with pigmentation and scarring temporal to the disc. A line scan shows a deep cavitary depression within the optic nerve that is significantly more exaggerated than what is seen in normal optic nerve cupping. There are associated hyporeflective cystic changes within the nerve fiber layer (arrow). There is shadowing due to overhanging of the nasal optic nerve rim with loss of the underlying OCT signal (arrowhead). The blue line (inset) shows the position of the B-scan.

Figure 6.3.2 (A) Color photograph of an optic nerve pit (arrow) previously treated with focal laser photocoagulation temporal to the optic disc. (B) Line scan shows intraretinal schisis of the outer nuclear layer (arrow). Chorioretinal atrophy, as a result of the prior laser treatment, can be seen (arrowheads). This OCT scan does not go through the optic nerve pit. (C) Line scan through an optic disc pit showing intraretinal schisis of the outer nuclear layer (arrow). The optic nerve pit can be seen in cross section (arrowheads).

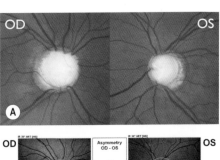

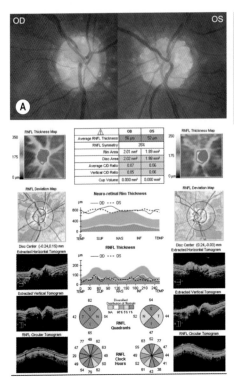

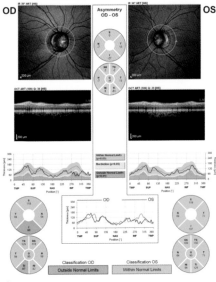

Figure 6.3.3 Color photograph of a patient with bilateral optic nerve head drusen. Note the elevated calcified deposits in the ONH of both right eye (RE) and left eye (LE). The retinal vessels that emerge from the ONH have normal appearance. ONH and RNFL analysis shows reduction in the average RNFL thickness in both eyes, and altered values of RNFL thickness measurement in fundus quadrants. The B-scan across the ONH reveals elevation and shadowing typical of ONH drusen.

Figure 6.3.4 Color photograph of a patient with bilateral megalopapilla shows enlarged optic disc area with increased cup-to-disc ratio. The cups are round and notching of the neuroretinal rim is not observed. SD-OCT shows increased optic disc area, 4.24 mm^2 and 2.75 mm^2 as measured by Heidelberg Retina Tomograph (Heidelberg Engineering GmbH, Heidelberg, Germany). Despite the increased cup-to-disc ratio and clinical diffuse absence of neuroretinal rim tissue in both eyes, the OCT showed normal RNFL thickness in the left eye (LE) and sectorial RNFL thinning only in the inferior sector in the right eye (RE). Of note, the normative data in the OCT software is valid for disc areas between 1.2 mm^2 and 2.8 mm^2, which might be related to the warning message in the right eye. *(Image courtesy of Dr Patricia Cerqueira, Sao Paulo University.)*

PART 3: Macular Disorders

7.1 | Dry Age-Related Macular Degeneration

Introduction: Dry age-related macular degeneration (AMD) accounts for a significant degree of visual disability in elderly populations. Loss of vision is secondary to photoreceptor cell death, which manifests clinically as geographic atrophy (GA). The dry form of AMD comprises approximately 85% of all AMD cases and currently has no available effective treatment.

Clinical Features: The hallmark feature of dry AMD is the presence of drusen, which are yellow-colored subretinal deposits that range in size and appearance (Fig. 7.1.1). Small, fine drusen without other manifestations such as RPE changes or atrophy should not be considered AMD. Additionally, there can be varied pigmentary changes within the RPE. Advanced forms of AMD feature atrophy of the RPE with eventual GA, which can occur in the presence or absence of drusen (Fig. 7.1.2 and Fig. 7.1.3).

OCT Features: **Drusen** are identified on OCT by their characteristic appearance as **discrete elevations of the RPE layer** at the level of Bruch's membrane (Figs. 7.1.4 and 7.1.5). Drusen may be of varying size and contour. Drusen can be described histopathologically as **basal linear**, when the deposits occur between the basement membrane of the RPE and Bruch's membrane (more typical), or **basal laminar**, when the deposits occur between the plasma membrane of the RPE and the basement membrane of the RPE. Basal laminar drusen are also called **cuticular** drusen and are characteristically small and regular shaped in a diffuse arrangement within the macula. It is difficult to distinguish between basal linear and basal laminar drusen on OCT. **GA** is identified by absence of the outer retinal layers and RPE, which leads to a **reverse shadowing effect** (Fig. 7.1.6).

Ancillary Testing: Color fundus photographs and fundus autoflourescence can be helpful to highlight and track areas of GA (Fig 7.1.3).

Treatment: No treatment is currently available for dry AMD though numerous research endeavors are underway, particularly for the treatment of GA.

FIGURE LEGENDS

Figure 7.1.1 Color fundus photograph of dry AMD with many drusen of varying size intermixed with RPE hyperpigmentation and hypopigmentation. There is an area of geographic atrophy (arrowheads), which is difficult to appreciate clinically.

Figure 7.1.2 Color fundus photograph of a large area of central geographic atrophy (arrowheads) and surrounding soft drusen.

Figure 7.1.3 Fundus autofluorescence image (corresponding to Figure 7.1.1) highlights areas of geographic atrophy as distinct areas of hypoautofluorescence.

Figure 7.1.4 OCT (corresponding to Figure 7.1.1) showing features of dry AMD. There are many discrete, round, hill-shaped elevations below the RPE, which are basal linear drusen (arrows). Drusen exhibit a medium-intensity

reflectance pattern on OCT. The choroidal thickness is typically less than normal in AMD (space between arrowheads).

Figure 7.1.5 OCT showing basal laminar or cuticular drusen. An associated pseudovitelliform detachment is present in the macula, which can be seen in the setting of cuticular drusen, even in the absence of choroidal neovascularization.

Figure 7.1.6 OCT (corresponding to Figure 7.1.2) showing larger (between arrows) and smaller (between arrowheads) areas of GA. In areas of GA, there is loss of the outer retinal layers and RPE. Due to absence of the RPE in these areas, the OCT signal is able to penetrate more deeply, which exaggerates the typical signal pattern so that there is a 'reverse' shadowing effect.

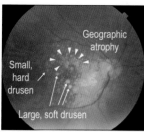

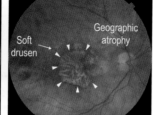

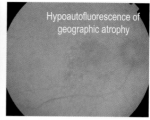

Figure 7.1.1

Figure 7.1.2

Figure 7.1.3

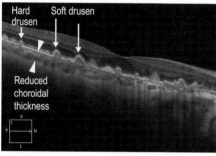

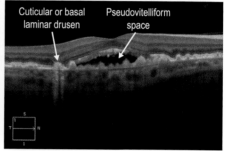

Figure 7.1.4

Figure 7.1.5

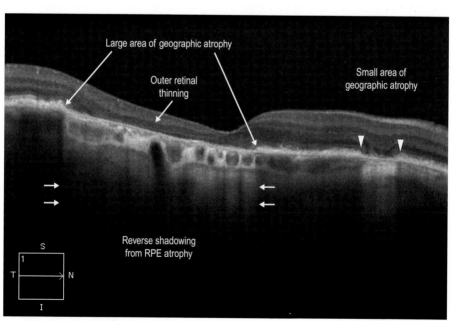

Figure 7.1.6

8.1 | Wet Age-Related Macular Degeneration

Introduction: Wet (neovascular, exudative) age-related macular degeneration (AMD) is a leading cause for severe vision loss in the elderly population of developed societies. It represents approximately 10% of all AMD cases.

Clinical Features: The distinguishing feature is the presence of choroidal neovascularization (CNV) in the setting of a patient over the age of 60 years, virtually always with some manifestations of concurrent or pre-existing dry AMD (drusen, geographic atrophy, RPE abnormalities). CNV results in leakage of fluid and/or hemorrhage within or underneath the neurosenory retina, and/or underneath the RPE detachment visible on examination. On the basis of fluorescein angiography, CNV can be subtyped into classic, occult, or mixed. An anatomic classification divides CNV into type 1 (below the RPE), type 2 (above the RPE) or type 3 (retinal angiomatosis proliferation [RAP]). In the presence of a large pigment epithelial detachment (PED), a tear of the RPE can occur. End-stage wet AMD may results in disciform scar formation.

OCT Features: The most characteristic findings on OCT in wet AMD are the presence of an **irregularly shaped PED** with adjacent **subretinal hemorrhage** and **subretinal fluid**. An irregularly shaped PED is in contrast to a more smooth-shaped PED typically seen in central serous chorioretinopathy. In wet AMD, especially in type 2 CNV, there is frequently a visible interruption in the RPE layer. There are various key features of wet AMD that can be uniquely identified based on their OCT appearance:

▸ **Classic CNV**: a classic, or type 2, CNV is present when the abnormal neovascular tissue penetrates the RPE/Bruch's membrane complex and is present in the subretinal space (Figs 8.1.1 and 8.1.2).

▸ **Occult CNV**: an occult, or type 1, CNV is present when the abnormal neovascular tissue remains underneath the RPE (Figs 8.1.3 and 8.1.4).

FIGURE LEGENDS

Figure 8.1.1 OCT of a classic choroidal neovascularization (far right). Corresponding thickness map (left) and infrared image (middle) are shown.

Figure 8.1.2 Fluorescein angiography (corresponding to Figure 8.1.1) shows a well-defined region of hyperfluorescence that is visible in the early frames and grows in intensity in the late frames, but does not enlarge in size, characteristic of a classic choroidal neovascularization (red circle).

Figure 8.1.3 Fluorescein angiography shows late hyperfluorescence with ill-defined boundaries, which may represent a fibrovascular pigment epithelial detachment, and is characteristic of an occult choroidal neovascularization (within red border).

Figure 8.1.4 OCT (corresponding to Figure 8.1.3) of an occult choroidal neovascularization (right) and corresponding thickness map (left), PED.

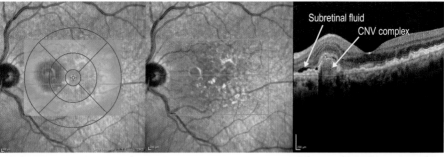

Figure 8.1.1

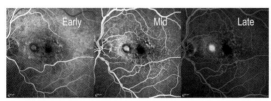

Figure 8.1.2

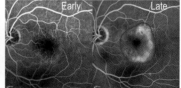

Figure 8.1.3

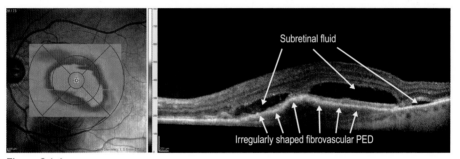

Figure 8.1.4

▸ **RPE tear**: an RPE tear has a very characteristic OCT appearance (Figs 8.1.5 and 8.1.6), where there is a sharply demarcated region of absent RPE adjacent to an area of bunched-up RPE.

▸ **Disciform scar**: a disciform scar can have a varied OCT appearance but always is dominated by a hyper-reflective subretinal scar (Figs 8.1.7 and 8.1.8).

FIGURE LEGENDS

Figure 8.1.5 OCT of a choroidal neovascularization with a large, irregular pigment epithelial detachment. The corresponding infrared image is also shown (left).

Figure 8.1.6 OCT of the same choroidal neovascularization shown in Figure 8.1.5 one month following treatment with intravitreal anti-VEGF therapy with resultant retinal pigment epithelium (RPE) tear. Due to the absence of the RPE in the region of the tear, reverse shadowing is seen in the deeper structures. The RPE is bunched up where it is still present, blocking deeper structures. There

is also still a thin rim of subretinal fluid present. Corresponding infrared image is shown on the left, which helps to visualize the region of the RPE tear.

Figure 8.1.7 Color photograph of a subretinal disciform scar that is the result of end-stage wet AMD. A central intraretinal cyst is present , which is better visualized on OCT.

Figure 8.1.8 OCT (corresponding to Figure 8.1.7) shows highly reflective subretinal material corresponding to the organized subretinal scar. A central intraretinal cyst is also present.

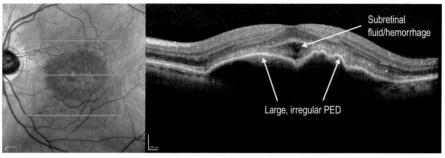

Figure 8.1.5

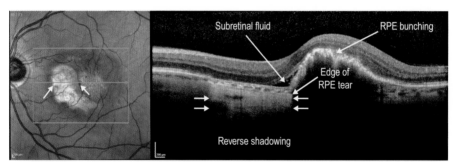

Figure 8.1.6

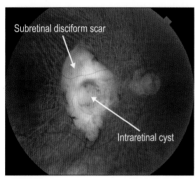

Figure 8.1.7

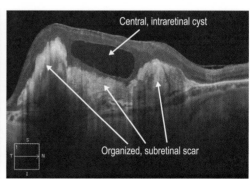

Figure 8.1.8

▸ **Treated CNV:** following treatment with anti-vascular endothelial growth factor (VEGF) therapy, intra- and subretinal fluid will often improve significantly or completely resolved (Figs 8.1.9 and 8.1.10). Associated PEDs also tend to decrease in size with continued treatment.

▸ **Retinal angiomatous proliferation:** type 3 CNV (or RAP), is a rare cause of exudative AMD resulting from abnormal neovascular tissue within the deep retina that typically originates within the retina and migrates towards the choriocapillaris and/or retinal surface (Figs 8.1.11 and 8.1.12).

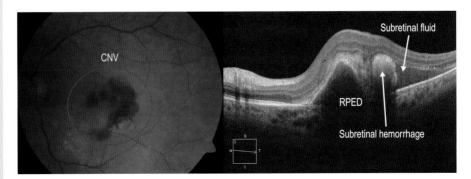

Figure 8.1.9 OCT shows all of the features of wet AMD including an irregularly shaped PED, subretinal hemorrhage, and subretinal fluid. Subretinal fluid lacks reflectivity on OCT and appears as an empty space, whereas the subretinal hemorrhage has moderate reflectivity and appears as a medium-intensity signal. The corresponding color photograph is shown on the left.

Figure 8.1.10 Following therapy with numerous intravitreal injections of an anti-vascular endothelial growth factor medication, there was significant improvement in the clinical appearance with resolution of subretinal fluid.

Figure 8.1.11 Color photograph of retinal angiomatous proliferation shows multiple localized intraretinal hemorrhages in an area of retinal thickening.

Figure 8.1.12 OCT (corresponding to Figure 8.1.10) shows a hyper-reflective area within the retina, thought to represent the retinal angiomatosis proliferation lesion. There is associated intraretinal cystic fluid and underlying subretinal fluid and pigment epithelial detachments.

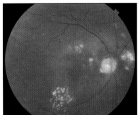

Figure 8.1.13

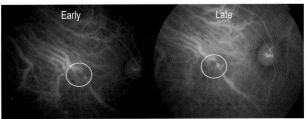

Figure 8.1.14

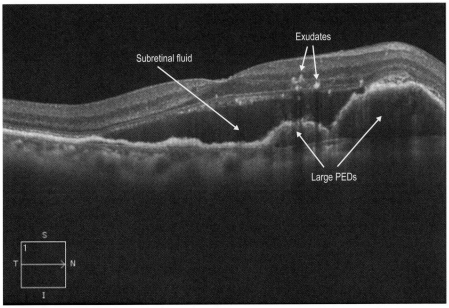

Figure 8.1.15

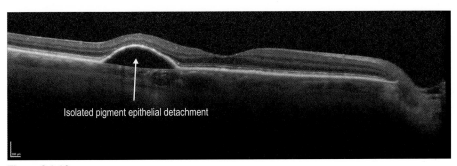

Figure 8.1.16

9.1 Posterior Staphyloma

Introduction: Posterior staphyloma occurs in the setting of high myopia (axial length >26 mm) as a result of progressive anteroposterior elongation of the globe over time with scleral thinning in the posterior pole.

Clinical Features: Externally, the globe itself may appear elongated, which is consistent with high myopia. On fundoscopy, there are associated atrophic changes of the retina, retinal pigment epithelium, and choroid in the posterior pole (Fig. 9.1.1). A teacup-like deformity is present, typically within the macula, but can also involve the optic nerve. The deformity can be difficult to appreciate clinically and requires stereopsis to appreciate.

OCT Features: The appearance of a posterior staphyloma on OCT is rather striking compared to the more subtle clinical appearance. OCT reveals significant **posterior bowing and curvature of the posterior eye wall,** including the sclera and overlying choroid and retinal layers (Fig. 9.1.2). The choroid is typically almost imperceptible due to significant thinning.

Ancillary Testing: Ultrasonography can be used to document progressive enlargement of the globe as well as to reveal the posterior out-pouching of the posterior wall of the eye.

Treatment: Treatment of any associated pathology may be required, but no primary therapy for the progressive globe enlargement has been proven to work.

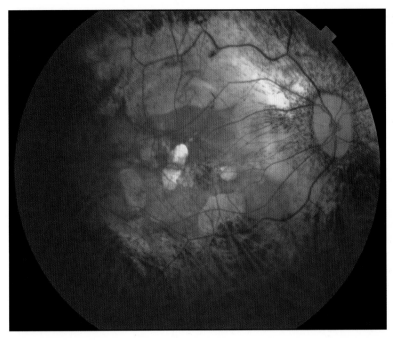

Figure 9.1.1 Color photograph of a posterior staphyloma involving the macula. There is extensive retinal pigment epithelium loss, pigmentary changes, and choroidal atrophy present.

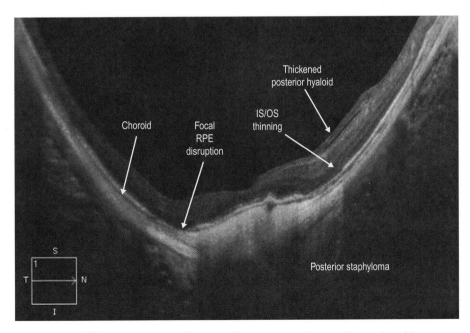

Figure 9.1.2 OCT (corresponding to Figure 9.1.1) shows dramatic posterior bowing of the eye wall. The choroid is so thin that it is barely appreciable. The RPE layer has focal disruptions. The retina takes on the same curvature as the sclera. There is also a mild dome-shaped macula present (see Chapter 9.4, Dome-Shaped Macula)

9.2 | Myopic Choroidal Neovascular Membrane

Introduction: Choroidal neovascular membrane (CNV) can occur in the setting of pathologic myopia, typically in pre-existing areas of Bruch's membrane weakness such as lacquer cracks and chorioretinal atrophy.

Clinical Features: This type of CNV is usually well-circumscribed, heavily pigmented, and in a background of typical myopic changes (Fig. 9.2.1). It typically involved the fovea and is a type 2, or classic, CNV subtype. Its behavior tends to be less aggressive than CNV associated with wet age-related macular degeneration.

OCT Features: Acutely, the CNV complex appears as a well-circumscribed area of **mixed reflectivity** in the subretinal space with overlying sub- and intraretinal fluid (Fig. 9.2.2, inset lower right). Sometimes, the presence of active CNV in high myopia **can be difficult to discern**, even with OCT. In this setting, activity may be recognized by **subtle changes on serial exams** (Figs 9.2.3 to 9.2.6). For such comparisons to be accurate, the scans that are taken at different times should be **registered** to assure the exact same region is being imaged over time. In the setting of myopic CNV, thickness maps are often fraught with segmentation artifact and cannot always be relied on to make treatment decisions.

Ancillary Testing: Fluorescein angiography (FA) can be helpful to confirm the presence of a type 2 CNV (Fig. 9.2.7).

Treatment: The mainstay of treatment is with intravitreal anti-VEGF therapy, with photodynamic therapy reserved for select cases.

FIGURE LEGENDS

Figure 9.2.1 Color photograph of a myopic CNV shows a well-circumscribed, darkly pigmented submacular lesion involving the inferior fovea.

Figure 9.2.2 A horizontal line scan OCT (corresponding to Figure 9.2.1) of the fovea shows thin subretinal fluid with overlying intraretinal fluid at the edge of the lesion. The corresponding thickness map (inset, upper right) helps identify the affected area of thickened retina. A vertical line scan OCT (inset, bottom right) shows an elevated subretinal lesion with mixed reflectivity corresponding to the CNV.

Figure 9.2.3 OCT shows a subretinal dome-shaped hyper-reflective area, which represents a myopic CNV. The distinction of the CNV from the overlying retina is blurred due to subretinal hemorrhage and subretinal fluid. These findings are more subtle in a myopic CNV in comparison to other forms of CNV. Characteristic myopic findings including a thin choroid and retinal schisis are also seen.

Figure 9.2.4 OCT (corresponding to Figure 9.2.3) shows a much more distinct border of the retina (arrowheads) and underlying myopic CNV one month following treatment with anti-VEGF therapy.

Figure 9.2.5 OCT of a small myopic CNV shows an ill-defined medium reflectivity subretinal elevation that obscures the photoreceptor and ELM layers and has poorly defined edges. *(Courtesy of Caroline Baumal, MD.)*

Figure 9.2.6 OCT (corresponding to Figure 9.2.5) shows complete resolution of the myopic CNV one month following treatment with intravitreal bevacizumab. *(Courtesy of Caroline Baumal, MD.)*

Figure 9.2.7 Fluorescein angiography (late phase, corresponding to Figure 9.2.1) shows a well-circumscribed area of hyperfluorescence consistent with a type 2 CNV.

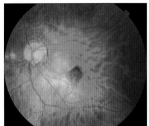

Figure 9.2.1

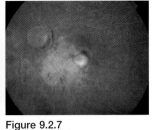

Figure 9.2.7

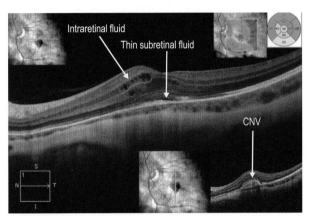

Intraretinal fluid

Thin subretinal fluid

CNV

Figure 9.2.2

Subretinal hemorrhage

Subretinal fluid

Myopic retinal schisis

CNV

Thin choroid

Figure 9.2.3

CNV

Figure 9.2.4

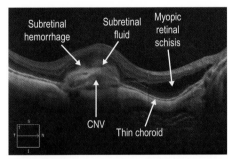

Small myopic CNV

Figure 9.2.5

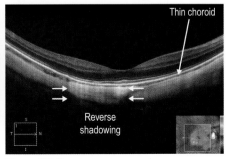

Thin choroid

Reverse shadowing

Figure 9.2.6

9.3 | Myopic Macular Schisis

Introduction: Myopic macular (foveal) schisis is a relatively common finding in eyes with high myopia and the prevalence increases with the degree of myopia. Mild cases do not necessarily impact visual acuity, whereas severe cases usually affect vision. Prior to the advent of OCT, this disorder was significantly under-recognized and poorly described.

Clinical Features: When mild, macular schisis is difficult, if not impossible to appreciate clinically. The presence of macular schisis in the setting of high myopia is usually only presumed based on the concomitant presence of other associated features of pathologic myopia such as posterior staphyloma, lacquer cracks, and atrophy. More severe cases can be recognized by the diffuse cystic change in the macula, presence of subretinal fluid or development of lamellar or full-thickness macular hole.

OCT Features: OCT is critical in confirming the diagnosis and following the morphologic changes in myopic schisis. OCT can readily visualize subtle schisis that is often asymptomatic (Fig. 9.3.1), and may be confused for other conditions such as cystoid macular edema. There is a characteristic **splitting of the retinal layers** that tends to occur in the **outer layers**, leaving a thicker inner retina split from a thinner outer retina. Joining these two layers are **perpendicular strands**, which may represent stretched Müller cells. There can be a range of severity in myopic macular schisis, including more moderate (Fig. 9.3.2) and severe (Fig. 9.3.3) changes. The choroid is characteristically thin, as in other instances of high myopia. Other changes include prominent posterior hyaloid, epiretinal membrane, lamellar macular hole or full-thickness macular hole.

Ancillary Testing: Fluorescein angiography is rarely helpful but can be used to rule out myopic choroidal neovascularization. B-scan ultrasonography can reveal some of the features but lacks the resolution of OCT.

Treatment: In mild to moderate cases, no treatment is warranted. However, in severe cases with progressive visual loss, vitrectomy can improve both the anatomy and the vision.

FIGURE LEGENDS

Figure 9.3.1 OCT of mild myopic macular schisis with splitting of the retina at the level of the outer nuclear layer and outer plexiform layer junction. The space created by the schisis is thickest centrally and tapers on each end, which is more apparent in other figures below.

Figure 9.3.2 OCT of moderate myopic macular schisis shows splitting of the retina within the inner portion of the outer nuclear layer. The central area of schisis is thickest with tapering on either side. Three-dimensionally, the schisis space would resemble a flying saucer. Within the schisis cavity, there are perpendicular strands crossing the full length of the cavity, which may represent Müller's cell footplates. Also note that there is a mild posterior staphyloma and dome-shaped macula present. The choroid is also characteristically thin.

Figure 9.3.3 OCT of severe myopic macular schisis shows dramatic splitting of the retina within the outer nuclear layer. Many perpendicular strands are crossing the schisis cavity. The choroid is almost not discernible due to significant thinning.

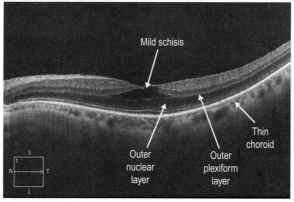

Figure 9.3.1

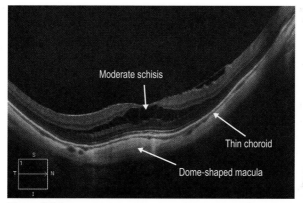

Figure 9.3.2

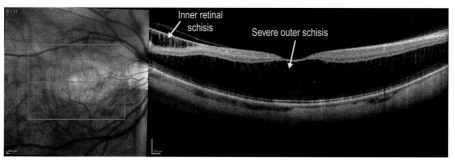

Figure 9.3.3

9.4 | Dome-Shaped Macula

Introduction: Dome-shaped macula is a rare recently identified finding in some highly myopic eyes. It is unclear why certain eyes are affected, but it seems to be due to localized variations in scleral thickness.

Clinical Features: There is an inward protuberance of the central macula within the larger concave shape of a posterior staphyloma in highly myopic eyes. This condition is not appreciated clinically and was only discovered with the advent of OCT.

OCT Features: A **vertical line scan** is more helpful than a horizontal scan in diagnosing dome-shaped macula. Within the convexity of a posterior staphyloma, there is an **inward bowing of the sclera** within the **central macula** (Fig. 9.4.1). The overlying macula follows the same contour as the sclera and there is often a **cap of subretinal fluid** (hyporeflective space), in the absence of any CNV or CSCR. The choroid is typically thin and the underlying sclera can usually be imaged well with standard spectral domain OCT protocols. However, both enhanced depth and swept source imaging techniques offer the ability to visualize deeper structures and are a better choice for assisting in this diagnosis, if available.

Ancillary Testing: Fluorescein can be helpful to rule out the presence of a concomitant CNV or CSCR.

Treatment: There is no treatment indicated. It is particularly important that, when present, the apparent cap of subretinal fluid is not anti-VEGF or photodynamic therapy responsive. It should not be considered as proof of the presence of a CNV. A brief anti-VEGF therapeutic trial can be considered, but is unlikely to be of benefit.

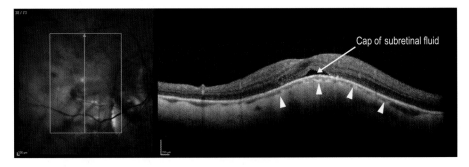

Cap of subretinal fluid

Figure 9.4.1 Vertical OCT line scan in dome-shaped macula shows characteristic inward protuberance of the sclera under the central macula (arrowheads). There is also a cap of hyporeflective subretinal fluid, which is present in the absence of choroidal neovascularization.

9.5 | Myopic Tractional Retinal Detachment

Introduction: In the presence of high myopia, a localized tractional retinal detachment within the macula is an uncommon occurrence. The underlying mechanism is not entirely clear, but tractional forces are thought to be the predominant factor.

Clinical Features: A localized elevation of the retina isolated to the macula is visible clinically in the absence of any visible, peripheral retinal breaks.

OCT Features: The presence of a large neurosensory detachment of the retina, isolated to the macula, is present (Fig. 9.5.1). There are often associated vitreous membranes with tractional insertions on the detachment. Other pathologic features of high myopia are usually present such as posterior staphyloma, macular schisis and/or macular hole.

Ancillary Testing: None.

Treatment: Initial observation may occasionally result in spontaneous release of vitreomacular traction with improvement in the retinal detachment. More commonly, surgical intervention is required with vitrectomy.

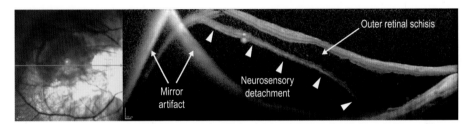

Figure 9.5.1 OCT of a myopic tractional retinal detachment shows a large neurosensory detachment of the retina (arrowheads). There is also significant overlying macular schisis and a posterior staphyloma. Towards the left side of the OCT, there is mirror artifact.

10.1 | Vitreomacular Adhesion and Vitreomacular Traction

Introduction: Vitreomacular adhesion (VMA) is an OCT finding. It represents a perifoveolar detachment of the cortical vitreous from the underlying retina with part of the vitreous remaining attached at the macula and elsewhere in the eye. The underlying macular retina is normal. It is almost always a normal finding, representing the initial evolution of a normal posterior vitreous detachment. Vitreomacular traction (VMT) is present when perifoveolar vitreous detachment is accompanied by retinal morphological changes arising from traction of the vitreous on the retina. There is no known racial predilection for VMT. VMT is more common in women (about 65%), with most patients in their sixth or seventh decade of life

Clinical Features: Patients may complain of decreased central vision with metamorphopsia. On examination, there may be preretinal fibrosis, epiretinal membrane formation and blunting or alteration of the foveal reflex with a pseudo-hole appearance.

OCT Diagnosis: OCT is the diagnostic modality of choice for both of these entities. In fact, VMA can *only* be reliably diagnosed via OCT. In VMA, OCT shows vitreous separating from around the macula with **persisting adhesion at the macular center**, often in a concentric fashion (Fig. 10.1.1). VMT is accompanied by changes in the retina including **cystic changes**, **macular schisis**, defined as a separation between the outer nuclear and the outer plexiform layer, **epiretinal membrane formation** and **tractional retinal detachment** (Figs 10.1.2 to 10.1.4) Often the posterior hyaloid appears **abnormally thickened** in VMT.

Ancillary Testing: A diagnosis of VMT is best made via OCT. Fluorescein angiography may show leakage in a cystic pattern. B-scan ultrasound may demonstrate peripheral detached vitreous, but with attachment still noted over the posterior pole.

Treatment: VMA should be observed. The term 'symptomatic VMA' will always appear as VMT on OCT. Mild VMT is typically observed. Surgery via vitrectomy or pharmacologic intervention can be considered for eyes with poor or worsening vision.

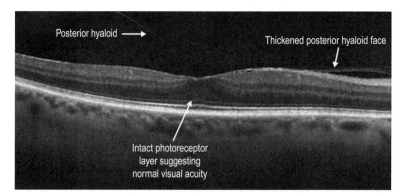

Figure 10.1.1 Vitreomacular adhesion. Note the dense posterior hyaloid face (arrows). The retina appears to be normal.

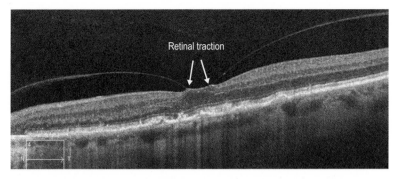

Figure 10.1.2 Early vitreomacular traction/stage 1 macular hole. The OCT shows an adherent vitreoretinal interface with retinal changes.

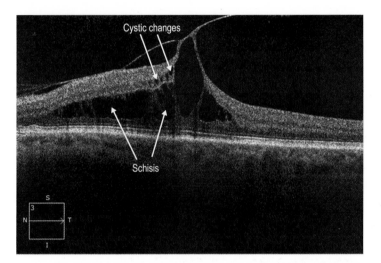

Figure 10.1.3 Vitreomacular traction with macular schisis and outer retinal cystic changes.

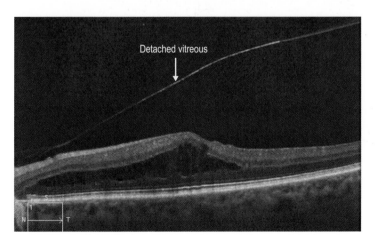

Figure 10.1.4 Vitreomacular traction post-treatment with ocriplasmin showing detachment of the vitreous over the macula (arrow) and improvement of the macular schisis.

10.2 | Full-Thickness Macular Hole

Introduction: A macular hole is a full-thickness defect in the neurosensory retina occurring at the macular center, usually associated with a central scotoma and decreased vision. Macular holes can be primary (formerly referred to as 'idiopathic'), resulting from vitreomacular traction (VMT) in the course of anomalous posterior vitreous detachment. Primary macular holes are more common in women, most often seen in the sixth or seventh decade of life. Primary macular holes may be bilateral in 10–20% of cases. Secondary macular holes are due to forces other than VMT. They can be traumatic, associated with posterior staphylomas in severe myopia, epiretinal membrane, cystoid macular edema, or rarely associated with solar retinopathy.

Clinical Features: Classic symptoms are acute unilateral decreased vision and occasional metamorphopsia. An impending macular hole may be seen as a loss of the normal fovelar depression with a yellow spot or ring in the center of the macula. A full-thickness macular hole (FTMH) is seen as a well demarcated, round red spot in the center of the macula surrounded by a grey halo that represents a cuff of subretinal fluid around the hole (Fig. 10.2.1) An operculum may be seen above the hole. Yellowish deposits may be seen within the hole.

Macular holes were classified according to their clinical findings. However, with OCT data available, this classification system is now in flux. This is described in some detail below.

OCT Features: OCT features of macular holes include a **full-thickness defect** in the neurosensory retina (Figs 10.2.2 to 10.2.4). There may be **cysts** in the neurosensory retina surrounding the area of the hole. A cuff of **subretinal fluid** may be seen around the defect in the retina. The vitreous may be attached to the hole with **vitreomacular traction** or there may be an **operculum** seen in the posterior vitreous on OCT scanning. Chronic macular holes may show loss of the cuff of subretinal fluid. There may also be **RPE atrophy** seen in chronic holes.

OCT-based macular hole classification is informed by the size of the hole and the status of the vitreomacular interface:

▸ **Stage 0 macular hole**: On OCT, this is an eye with VMA which has a FTMH in the contralateral eye. The risk of progression to a full-thickness hole in the eye with VMA may be close to 40%.
▸ **Stage 1 macular hole**: This is an eye with vitreomacular traction.
▸ **Stage 2, 3 and 4 macular holes** per Gass's classification are now re-classified as small, medium or large macular holes with (stage 4) or without (stage 2 and 3) release of the vitreomacular adhesion.

FTMHs are now better classified according to their aperture size on OCT scanning as measured by the caliper function of the OCT scanner:

▸ **Small FTMH** – aperture size less than or equal to 250 μm
▸ **Medium-sized FTMH** – aperture size between 250 μm and 400 μm
▸ **Large FTMH** – aperture size greater than 400 μm

FTMH may further be sub-classified by presence or absence of ongoing VMT.

Ancillary Testing: The diagnosis of a macular hole is made on examination and OCT scanning. Additional tests are usually not warranted

Management: For stage 0 and 1 macular holes, the management is as described in the VMA/VMT section (Chapter 10.1). FTMHs are typically treated surgically, with excellent prognosis for closure and visual recovery for small and intermediate sized holes. Chronic (>2 years) holes show slightly lower closure rate with surgery, but the visual results are significantly less than acute FTMH. Small and medium-sized FTMH can be treated with intravitreal ocriplasmin with closure rates of approximately 50%.

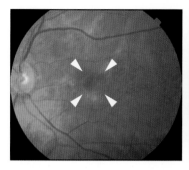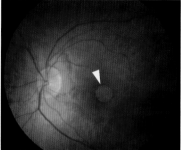

Figure 10.2.1 Fundus photograph of a full-thickness macular hole. The picture to the left shows an acute hole, whereas the one on the right shows a chronic hole with retinal pigment epithelium changes at the margin.

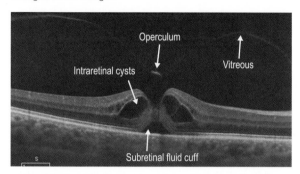

Figure 10.2.2 OCT scan through an acute macular hole showing intraretinal cysts, a cuff of subretinal fluid and an operculum . Note that the vitreous is detached from the fovea.

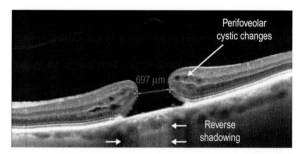

Figure 10.2.3 A large sized macular hole with the calipers showing a measurement of over 600 μm.

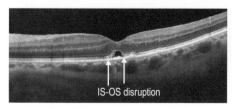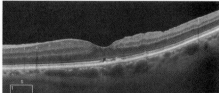

Figure 10.2.4 One week and one month post-vitrectomy for macular hole closure. Note the small area of subretinal elevation that decreases with time with restoration of the ELM and a small area of disruption in the IS–OS/ellipsoid layer. Various studies have shown that disruption in the ELM, IS–OS/ellipsoid layer, as well as the length of disruption of the cone outer segment tips correlates with level of post-operative visual acuity.

10.3 | Epiretinal Membrane

Introduction: Epiretinal membrane (ERM) affects 6% of patients over 60 years of age. They are most commonly due to vitreoschisis after posterior vitreous detachment, or associated with retinal tears and breaks, cryopexy, previous retinal laser, intraocular surgery, uveitis, or a history of trauma.

Clinical Features: Patients may be asymptomatic or complain of metamorphopsia and blurring of varying severity. On examination, the epiretinal layer can be seen as a glistening membrane overlying the fovea, often associated with retinal striae in a radial fashion and macular thickening (Fig. 10.3.1). Contraction of the membranes can also cause retinal vascular distortion. More severe epiretinal membranes can cause loss of the normal foveal reflex and 'pseudohole' formation.

OCT Features: ERM appears as a **highly reflective layer** overlying the inner retina, which may be adherent to the retina throughout the length of the scan, or **adherent** for only a portion of the macular region. Depending on the severity of the ERM, **distortion of the inner retina, loss of foveal contour, retinal thickening and irregularity of the retinal surface, subretinal fluid and foveal schisis** may occur (Figs 10.3.2 and 10.3.3). **Cystic changes** may also be seen within the retina. Occasionally, ERM may be associated with a **pseudohole** configuration, with **disruption** of the inner retina in the region of the 'hole' and **separation** between the outer plexiform layer and the outer nuclear layer seen adjacent to the site of the 'hole'. However, the outer retinal structures are intact including the inner and outer segments of the photoreceptors.

Ancillary Testing: Fluorescein angiography may highlight distortion of the blood vessels with leakage of blood vessels at the macula.

Treatment: The treatment of epiretinal membranes is either observation or surgery when the ERM starts to affect vision.

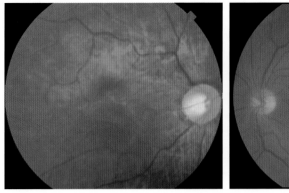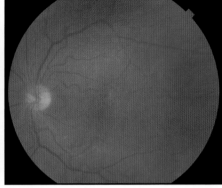

Figure 10.3.1 The photo on the right shows a mild epiretinal membrane with retinal striae. The photo on the left shows a more dense epiretinal membrane.

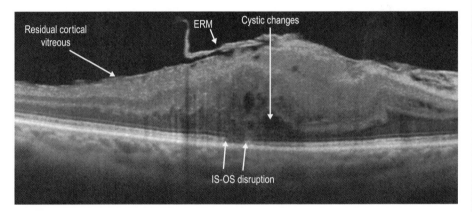

Figure 10.3.2 More dense ERM with macular edema, cystic changes, and distortion in the retinal architecture.

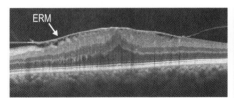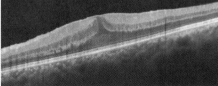

Figure 10.3.3 Preoperative and postoperative OCT scans through an epiretinal membrane (ERM). In the first figure, notice the hyper-reflective membrane causing macular edema. In the second image, the macular thickening is still present but the ERM has been removed.

11.1 | Postoperative Cystoid Macular Edema

Introduction: Postoperative cystoid macular edema (PCME) is a common cause of vision loss after surgery that can occur following virtually any intraocular procedure, including cataract surgery, vitrectomy, and glaucoma filtering surgery.

Clinical Features: PCME has the characteristic clinical appearance of numerous small cystic cavities bunched together in a petalloid arrangement centered on the fovea (Fig. 11.1.1, left). In some cases, the optic disc will be hyperemic or even frankly edematous. Small flame, shaped superficial hemorrhages in the inner retina are not rare.

OCT Features: The characteristic feature on OCT is **large, hyporeflective cystic spaces** located in the **outer plexiform layer**, though there can also be additional, smaller hyporeflective spaces within the inner plexiform and nuclear layers (Fig. 11.1.1, right). In severe cases, there may be a central neurosensory detachment. Following successful treatment, the cystic spaces seen on OCT typically improve (Fig. 11.1.2).

Ancillary Testing: In all cases, fluorescein angiography reveals PCME, even occasionally when it is not visible clinically or by OCT. The angiographic appearance is very characteristic with late diffuse central leakage in a petalloid pattern (Fig. 11.1.3).

Treatment: PCME is often a self-limited disease, but in visually significant cases various treatments can be used including topical therapy with corticosteroids and non-steroidal anti-inflammatory drugs, local corticosteroids, anti-vascular endothelial growth factors, or even vitrectomy.

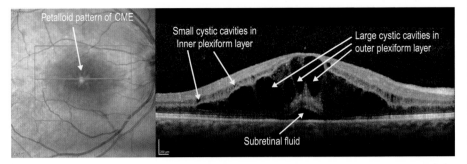

Figure 11.1.1 Infrared image (left) shows a petalloid arrangement of cystic cavities centered on the fovea, characteristic of PCME. OCT (right) shows numerous, hyporeflective cystic cavities located within the outer plexiform layer. There are also smaller hyporeflective cystic cavities located within the inner plexiform and inner nuclear layers. Subretinal fluid is present underneath the fovea. The outer nuclear layer located just above this fluid is hyper-reflective, which is likely an artifact due to the directional manner by which light traverses through the overlying large cystic cavities. *(Courtesy of Jeffrey S. Heier, MD.)*

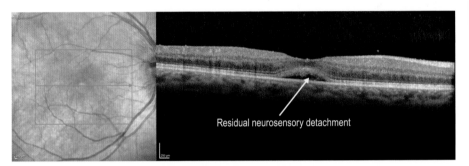

Figure 11.1.2 One month following treatment with topical anti-inflammatory agents, OCT show that the PCME is mostly resolved, though a small neurosensory detachment still remains. *(Courtesy of Jeffrey S. Heier, MD.)*

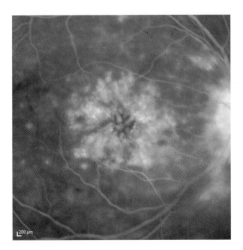

Figure 11.1.3 Fluorescein angiography shows florid late diffuse angiographic leakage in a petalloid pattern. The optic nerve is also leaking, which is not uncommon in severe PCME. *(Courtesy of Jeffrey S. Heier, MD.)*

11.2 | Macular Telangiectasia

Introduction: Macular telangiectasia (MacTel) is classified as type 1 or type 2. Type 1 MacTel is considered a form of Coats' disease and is developmental in origin. It is usually unilateral. Type 2 MacTel is an acquired, bilateral disorder that occurs in middle-aged or older adults.

Clinical Features: Type 1 MacTel is typically unilateral and features aneurysmal dilatations of capillaries within the macula. Surrounding exudates are common (Fig. 11.2.1). Type 2 MacTel is typically bilateral and features a loss of the temporal juxtafoveal retinal transparency followed by the development of ectatic capillaries in this region (Fig. 11.2.2). Over time, RPE hyperplasia and pigment deposition may occur along with crystal deposits (Fig. 11.2.3).

OCT Features
▶ MacTel type 1: there is cystoid **intraretinal edema** similar in appearance to cystoid macular edema from other etiologies (Fig. 11.2.4).

FIGURE LEGENDS

Figure 11.2.1 Color photograph of MacTel type 1 shows numerous aneurysmal abnormalities of varying size within the temporal macula. There is associated retinal thickening and surrounding hard exudate. The fellow macula was normal in appearance.

Figure 11.2.2 Color photograph of MacTel type 2 shows loss of the foveal reflex with subtle microaneurysmal abnormalities in the temporal parafoveal region. Fine, crystalline deposits in the same region are barely discernable, but could be seen clinically. Similar findings were seen in the fellow eye.

Figure 11.2.3 Color photograph of more advanced MacTel type 2 shows retinal pigment epithelium clumping and hyperplasia along with foveal atrophy and obvious crystalline deposits.

Figure 11.2.4 (A) OCT (corresponding to Figure 11.2.1) in MacTel type 1 shows numerous intraretinal cystic cavities of low and medium reflectivity and small hyperreflective deposits within the retina, corresponding to hard exudates. (B) OCT four months following treatment with focal grid laser shows a significant reduction in the cystoid macular edema and hard exudates. There are multiple discontinuous areas in the IS–OS/ellipsoid zone (arrowheads), which represent laser scars. (C) OCT two and a half years following focal laser treatment (no additional treatment was performed) shows resolution of cystoid macular edema with a small amount of residual exudate. The laser scars have faded (arrowhead).

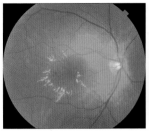

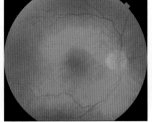

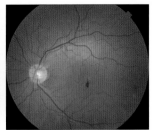

Figure 11.2.1

Figure 11.2.2

Figure 11.2.3

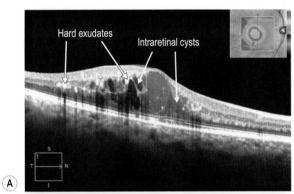

A

Hard exudates

Intraretinal cysts

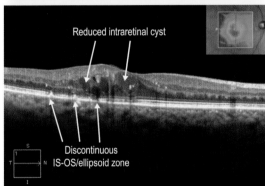

B

Reduced intraretinal cyst

Discontinuous
IS-OS/ellipsoid zone

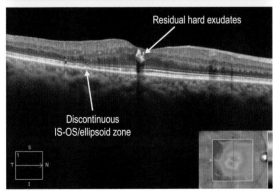

C

Residual hard exudates

Discontinuous
IS-OS/ellipsoid zone

Figure 11.2.4

▸ MacTel type 2: there are **lamellar defects within various layers** of the retina, characteristically involving the region just **temporal to the fovea,** which are seen on OCT as irregular, **hyporeflective cavities** (Fig. 11.2.5). These hyporeflective cavities can have varying appearances (Fig. 11.2.6), though the region temporal to the fovea rather than nasal is more involved. With chronic disease, pigment deposition and atrophy may develop (Fig. 11.2.7). Rarely, a secondary CNV can also occur (Fig. 11.2.8).

FIGURE LEGENDS

Figure 11.2.5 OCT (corresponding to Figure 11.2.2) in MacTel type 2 shows numerous hyporeflective cavities throughout multiple retinal layers, but limited to the temporal parafoveal region.

Figure 11.2.6 OCT in MacTel type 2 shows loss of tissue from the outer nuclear layer within the fovea, leaving hyporeflective cystic cavities, more prominent temporally. There is also underlying photoreceptor atrophy (arrowhead).

Figure 11.2.7 OCT (corresponding to Figure 11.2.3) in MacTel type 2 shows significant photoreceptor and retinal pigment epithelium (RPE) atrophy (between arrowheads). There is pigment migration from the RPE within the layers of the retina. A small hyporeflective cavity is present within the fovea. The crystalline deposits are not clearly seen.

Figure 11.2.8 (A) OCT in MacTel type 2 with characteristic hyporeflective intraretinal cavities involving the fovea, prior to the development of a CNV. (B) OCT at a later time point shows a CNV with adjacent subretinal fluid, which developed spontaneously.

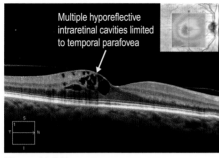

Figure 11.2.5

Multiple hyporeflective intraretinal cavities limited to temporal parafovea

Loss of tissue from outer nuclear layer leaving hyporeflective cavities

Photoreceptor atrophy

Figure 11.2.6

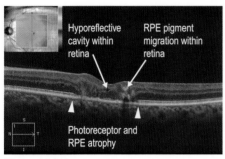

Hyporeflective cavity within retina

RPE pigment migration within retina

Photoreceptor and RPE atrophy

Figure 11.2.7

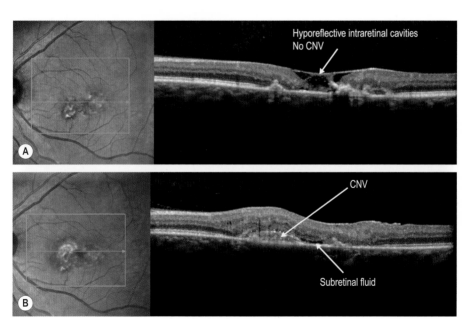

Hyporeflective intraretinal cavities No CNV

CNV

Subretinal fluid

Figure 11.2.8

Ancillary Testing: Fluorescein angiography can be helpful in both types of MacTel. In MacTel type 1, there are aneurysms of varying size and distribution associated with an abnormal capillary plexus or areas of non-perfusion (Fig. 11.2.9). In MacTel type 2, there are prominent telangiectatic capillaries in the temporal parafoveal region, which leak (Fig. 11.2.10). The cystic changes seen on OCT do not have corresponding leakage on FA. The FA changes may come before or after OCT evidence of the disease is present.

Treatment: There are no proven directed therapies toward MacTel type I but focal laser, photodynamic therapy, intravitreal corticosteroids, and anti-vascular endothelial growth factor have all been used. Secondary consequences such as choroidal neovascularization or macular hole in type 2 may require directed therapy.

FIGURE LEGENDS

Figure 11.2.9 FA (corresponding to Figure 11.2.1) shows numerous hyper-fluorescent aneurysmal capillary dilatations within an abnormal capillary network, most prominent in the temporal parafoveal region.

Figure 11.2.10 Fluorescein angiography (corresponding to Figure 11.2.2) shows an enlarged foveal avascular zone bordered by leaking capillary abnormalities in the temporal parafoveal region.

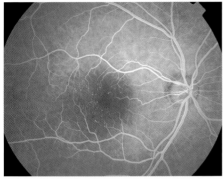

Figure 11.2.9

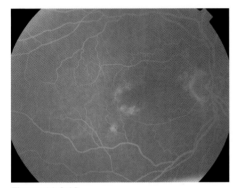

Figure 11.2.10

11.3 Uveitis

Introduction: Intermediate and posterior forms of uveitis both commonly affect posterior structures of the eye. Anterior uveitis can also occasionally cause cystoid macular edema (CME).

Clinical Features: Clinical findings vary widely depending on the specific disease state. Common symptoms include decreased vision, floaters, and a red, painful eye. Intraocular inflammation is the key finding. The primary location of intraocular inflammation determines whether anterior, intermediate, or posterior uveitis is present. Optic disc edema and CME may be associated clinical findings.

OCT Features: The presence of **optic disc edema**, **CME**, **subretinal fluid**, and **vitritis** are clinical features of uveitis that can be well visualized with OCT. Active sarcoid posterior uveitis can lead to optic disc edema, CME, and subretinal fluid (Fig. 11.3.1). OCT is useful in this setting to **monitor for treatment response** (Fig. 11.3.2). Sarcoid anterior uveitis can also result in isolated CME, which can sometimes be more readily detected on an **OCT thickness map** rather than a line scan (Fig. 11.3.3). Pars planitis often leads to associated CME (Fig. 11.3.4), which can respond well to treatment with periocular steroids (Fig. 11.3.5).

Ancillary Testing: A thorough, focused medical workup is often indicated in the setting of intermediate and posterior uveitis. Referral to a rheumatologist and/or uveitis specialist may be required in more complicated cases.

Treatment: Topical, periocular, and intravitreal steroids are the mainstay of local therapy. Systemic therapy with steroids or immunomodulators may be required via oral and/or intravenous routes.

FIGURE LEGENDS

Figure 11.3.1 OCT in a case of sarcoid posterior uveitis. Optic disc edema, cystoid macular edema, and subretinal fluid are present. The posterior hyaloid can be seen (arrowheads). The associated thickness map (inset) artifactually picks up the subretinal fluid as retinal thickness due to an error in the segmentation algorithm, which measures from the retinal pigment epithelium layer instead of the most posterior retina structure.

Figure 11.3.2 OCT three months following treatment with oral steroids (corresponding to Figure 11.3.1) shows resolution of the optic disc edema, cystoid macular edema, and subretinal fluid. Due to the segmentation error, the associated thickness map (inset) is useful to monitor improvement over time.

Figure 11.3.3 OCT in a case of sarcoid anterior uveitis shows subtle cystoid macular edema (CME), which was clinically symptomatic. The associated thickness map (inset) shows generalized parafoveal thickening, which gives a better overall sense of the CME than the isolated line scan. There is a strand of hyaloid that is visible, which is not of any clinical significance.

Figure 11.3.4 OCT in a case of pars planitis shows severe CME with associated subretinal fluid. The CME is located within the inner nuclear layer (red arrow) and Henle fiber layer (or axonal outer plexiform layer; white arrow). There is also a mild associated ERM.

Figure 11.3.5 OCT one month following treatment with sub-Tenons triamcinolone (corresponding to Figure 11.3.4) shows complete resolution of cystoid macular edema and subretinal fluid. The associated thickness map (inset) highlights these changes.

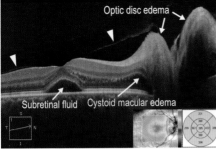

Figure 11.3.1

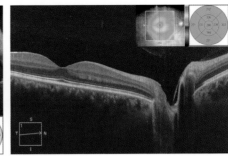

Figure 11.3.2

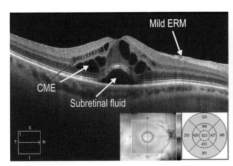

Figure 11.3.3

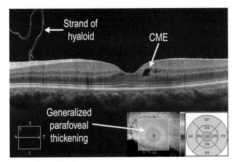

Figure 11.3.4

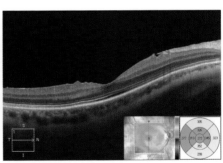

Figure 11.3.5

12.1 | Central Serous Chorioretinopathy

Introduction: Central serous chorioretinopathy is characterized in the acute phase by serous detachment of the retina over one or more areas of leakage from the choroid through a defect in the RPE. It is usually self-resolving, but rarely can become chronic. Its chronic phase is marked by retinal thinning, cystic retinal degeneration, cystoid macular edema, and diffuse RPE loss. This condition occurs most commonly in men between 20–50 years of age. Predisposing factors are type A personality, stressful events, corticosteroid use and conditions associated with hypercortisolism such as pregnancy and Cushing's disease.

Clinical Features: Patients usually present with a unilateral decrease and distortion of central vision. Examination reveals a macular, well-circumscribed neurosensory retinal detachment often with one or more retinal pigment epithelial detachments. Often signs of CSCR can also be found in the contralateral eye (Fig. 12.1.1).

OCT Features
- **Acute:** the OCT reveals a well-circumscribed neurosensory **retinal detachment** seen as an elevation of the retinal layers with **optically clear fluid** occupying the space between the outer retina and the RPE layer (Fig. 12.1.2). Often (75%) these are also associated with a small **pigment epithelial detachment**, seen as elevation of the RPE layer with underlying shadowing. The retina may sometimes be **thickened** in the acute phase. Choroidal thickening is usually noted compared to normal as well as to fellow eyes in acute CSCR, and this may be better visualized using the EDI protocol on most commercial OCT scanners. This **diffuse thickening** may be seen to improve when the acute phase of the CSCR resolves.
- **Chronic** CSCR may be accompanied by accumulation of hyper-reflective material in the subretinal space (Fig. 12.1.3). Cystic retinal changes and eventual retinal thinning has been reported overlying the areas of subretinal fluid in chronic CSCR. This may be accompanied by photoreceptor and RPE loss. The loss of photoreceptors on OCT may also be associated with decreased best corrected visual acuity even after resolution of subretinal fluid.
- **Multifocal** CSCR is characterized by multiple discrete areas of neurosensory detachments. As the CSCR resolves, the subretinal fluid is seen to decrease and then disappear. Quantitative OCT measurements of subretinal fluid are useful in monitoring for improvement and resolution.

Ancillary Testing: Fluorescein angiography shows one or more focal leaks at the RPE level with subretinal pooling of dye. Indocyanine green angiography, although usually not necessary to make the diagnosis, reveals large hyperfluorescent patches with late leakage. Fundus autofluorescence may show patchy areas of autohyperfuorescence in the macular area.

Treatment: Most cases of CSCR resolve spontaneously within 4–6 months with improvement of visual acuity. Occasionally, therapeutic options such as focal laser to the leaking spot or photodynamic therapy may be useful to expedite resolution or in chronic CSCR.

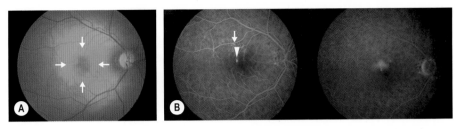

Figure 12.1.1 (A) Fundus photo showing a discrete, well-circumscribed elevation at the macula (arrows). (B) Fluorescein angiography in the early phase shows an area of hyperfluorescence (arrowhead) with leakage noted in the late phase. Note the adjacent areas of hyperfluorescence (arrow) indicative of RPE window defects characteristically seen in patients with central serous chorioretinopathy.

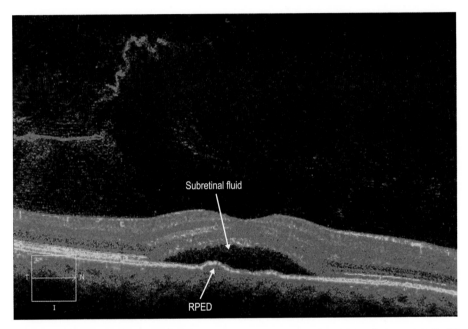

Figure 12.1.2 OCT scanning shows a neurosensory retinal detachment. A small pigment epithelial detachment can sometimes be visualized.

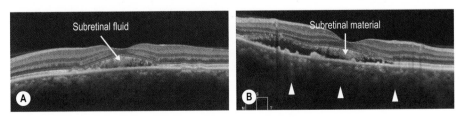

Figure 12.1.3 (A) Chronic central serous chorioretinopathy. Note the subretinal material accumulation and the change in reflectivity of the outer nuclear layer on OCT. (B) Enhanced depth imaging of chronic CSCR. Note that the bottom of the choroid cannot be visualized because of choroidal thickening (arrowheads). There is accumulation of subretinal material.

12.2 | Hydroxychloroquine Toxicity

Introduction: Retinal toxicity from hydroxychloroquine is rare, especially when dosed appropriately (≤6.5 mg/kg/day is recommended). After five years of use, the incidence is about 1% and increases with additive use over time. Patients with short stature and liver dysfunction appear to be at greater risk.

Clinical Features: The findings of hydroxychloroquine retinopathy, even in early and moderate disease, can be clinically silent. Later in the disease, there is a bull's eye maculopathy that becomes evident (Fig. 12.2.1).

OCT Features: OCT is one of the most useful and sensitive diagnostic tests for identifying retinal toxicity due to hydroxychloroquine. Findings in early disease can be very subtle and may only show up clearly on a retinal thickness map (Fig. 12.2.2). In moderate disease, there is more obvious **thinning of the outer retinal layers** in a **parafoveal** distribution including loss of the **retinal pigment epithelium (RPE) and IS/OS/ellipsoid zone** (Fig. 12.2.3). With advanced disease, there can be profound outer retinal layer loss in a **parafoveal wreath pattern** leading to a **flying saucer-like appearance** (Fig. 12.2.4). The **central fovea is characteristically preserved** even in advanced disease.

Ancillary Testing: Multifocal electroretinogram testing is very helpful in early or borderline cases to detect subtle abnormalities in central visual function. Fundus autofluorescence and central visual field testing (10–2) are also helpful as adjunctive tests.

Treatment: Stopping hydroxychloroquine at the earliest sign of retinal toxicity is crucial. Retinopathy is irreversibly and retinal toxicity may be progressive for some time period, even after discontinuation of hydroxychloroquine.

FIGURE LEGENDS

Figure 12.2.1 Color photograph of advanced hydrochloroquine retinopathy with a classic bull's eye maculopathy.

Figure 12.2.2 OCT in a patient with very early hydrochloroquine retinopathy shows an essentially normal line scan. The key finding is on the thickness map (inset), which reveals mild retinal thinning in a parafoveal pattern, more in the temporal macula.

Figure 12.2.3 OCT in a patient with moderate to advanced hydrochloroquine retinopathy shows fairly extensive outer retinal thinning with loss of the RPE and IS/OS/ellipsoid zone, particularly temporally (to right of arrowhead). There is also outer retinal loss to a milder degree in the nasal macula with early RPE and IS/OS/ellipsoid zone disruption. The corresponding thickness map (inset) nicely illustrates the degree of overall thinning.

Figure 12.2.4 OCT in a patient with advanced hydrochloroquine retinopathy (corresponding to Fig. 12.2.1) shows outer retinal thinning with abrupt dropout of the RPE and IS/OS/ellipsoid zone in a parafoveal ring (between arrowheads). There is a classic 'flying saucer' appearance due to preservation of the central fovea. The bull's eye maculopathy is seen on the corresponding OCT image (inset, left) and the degree of overall thinning is seen on the corresponding thickness map (inset, right).

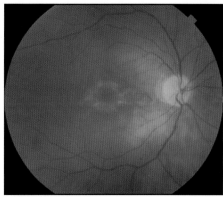

Figure 12.2.1

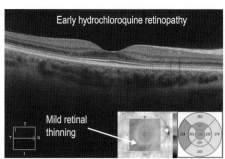

Early hydrochloroquine retinopathy

Mild retinal thinning

Figure 12.2.2

Moderate to advanced hydrochloroquine retinopathy

Significant outer retinal thinning

Early RPE and IS/OS/ellipsoid zone disruption

Figure 12.2.3

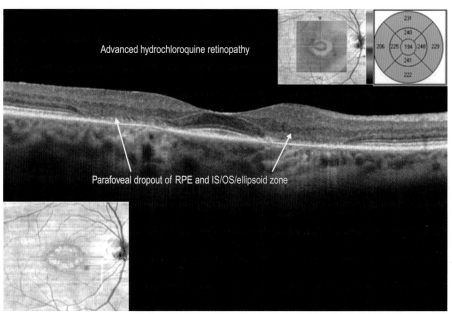

Advanced hydrochloroquine retinopathy

Parafoveal dropout of RPE and IS/OS/ellipsoid zone

Figure 12.2.4

12.3 Pattern Dystrophy

Introduction: Pattern dystrophies encompass a group of phenotypically similar macular disorders that are inheritable and share a common genetic defect in the *PRPH2* gene. They are usually inherited in an autosomal dominant pattern.

Clinical Features: There are dark, yellow, and/or orange pigment disturbances at the level of the RPE, leading to characteristic patterns of deposition in the central macula, which are often vitelliform-like (Fig. 12.3.1). There is a lifetime risk up to 18% of developing secondary choroidal neovascularization. The clinical features are usually symmetric, but there can be heterogeneity between eyes (Fig. 12.3.2).

OCT Features: A disturbance at the **level of the RPE** is the rule. In the setting of a **vitelliform-like lesion**, there is moderately reflective material underneath or within the RPE layer (Fig. 12.3.3). Below this are highly reflective, drusen-like deposits. In the absence of a vitelliform-like lesion, there are typically **highly reflective, drusen-like deposits** within the RPE layer (Fig. 12.3.4). There can be a **hyporeflective, empty space** overlying the pigmentary disturbance. The significance of this fluid-like compartment is not clearly understood, but it usually does not represent the presence of choroidal neovascularization and would not be expected to be VEGF-responsive.

Ancillary Testing: Fluorescein angiography can be helpful in ruling out secondary choroidal neovascularization, particularly when OCT reveals the presence of a fluid-like subretinal compartment. Fundus autofluorescence often has a characteristic appearance that can aid in the diagnosis (Fig. 12.3.5).

Treatment: No treatment is available, unless there is secondary choroidal neovascularization, which is treated with intravitreal anti-VEGF therapy.

FIGURE LEGENDS

Figure 12.3.1 Color fundus photograph shows a yellowish, circular vitelliform-like lesion within the central macula.

Figure 12.3.2 Color fundus photograph of fellow eye from Figure 12.3.1, shows numerous clumps of pigment within the central macula. This likely represents a collapsed vitelliform lesion.

Figure 12.3.3 OCT (corresponding to Figure 12.3.1) shows moderately reflective material that appears to split the RPE layer. There are also highly reflective, drusen-like deposits underlying this area.

Figure 12.3.4 OCT (corresponding to Figure 12.3.2) shows highly reflective, drusen-like deposits corresponding to the pigment disturbances seen in the color photograph.

Figure 12.3.5 Fundus autofluorescence shows a well-circumscribed, circular area of hyperautofluorescence with inter-mingled, splotchy, small areas of hypoautofluorescence.

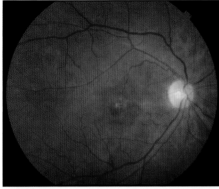

Figure 12.3.2

Figure 12.3.1

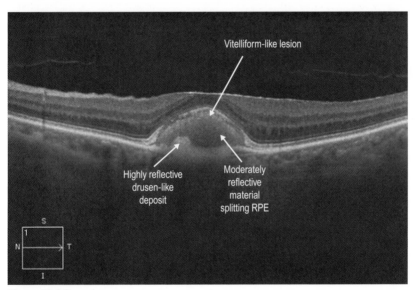

Figure 12.3.3

Vitelliform-like lesion

Highly reflective
drusen-like
deposit

Moderately
reflective
material
splitting RPE

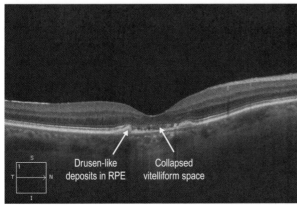

Figure 12.3.4

Drusen-like
deposits in RPE

Collapsed
vitelliform space

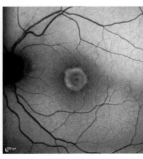

Figure 12.3.5

12.4 Oculocutaneous Albinism

Introduction: Oculocutaneous albinism is a rare, typically autosomal recessive, disorder featuring a dysfunction of the melanin producing cells in the eye, hair, and skin. Tyrosinase-negative forms feature an inability to produce melanin, whereas tyrosinase-positive forms have a decreased ability to produce melanin.

Clinical Features: The fundus of tyrosinase-negative individuals have a complete lack of pigmentation, whereas tyrosinase-positive individuals have a variable, but reduced, amount of fundus pigmentation (Fig. 12.4.1). Foveal hypoplasia is characteristically present in both types.

OCT Features: OCT line scans of the central macula reveal **lack of a distinguished foveal depression**, evidence of foveal hypoplasia (Fig. 12.4.2). As a result of this, the corresponding thickness map shows central 'thickening' in comparison to the normative database.

Ancillary Testing: Abnormal decussation of temporal nerve fibers is a characteristic feature seen on visually evoked cortical potential testing. Genetic testing can be performed for mutations in the four genes (*TYR*, *OCA2*, *TYRP1*, or *SLC45A2*) which, when defective, cause different forms of the disease.

Treatment: Chediak–Higashi and Hermansky–Pudlak syndromes are associated with oculocutaneous syndrome and can be lethal. Frequent infections may be seen in Chediak–Higashi syndrome and easy bruising can be seen in Hermansky–Pudlak syndrome. Prompt hematologic consultation should be made if either of these syndromes is suspected.

FIGURE LEGENDS

Figure 12.4.1 Color photograph of a patient with tyrosinase-positive oculocutaneous albinism shows a blond fundus with no distinct fovea.

Figure 12.4.2 OCT line scan (corresponding to Figure 12.4.1) through the central macula shows foveal hypoplasia with lack of a well-defined foveal depression. The accompanying thickness map (inset) shows increased thickness centrally in comparison to a normative database due to the lack of a normal foveal depression.

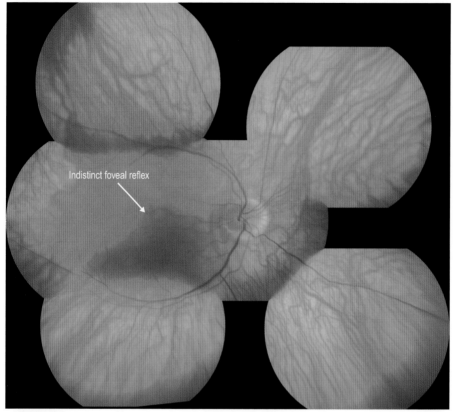

Figure 12.4.1

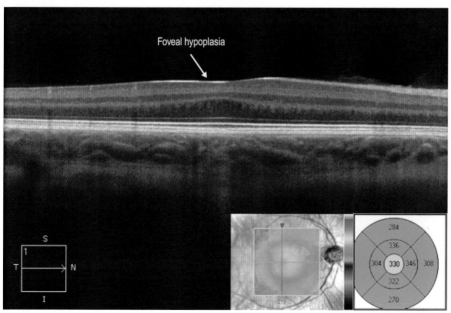

Figure 12.4.2

12.5 Subretinal Perfluorocarbon

Introduction: Perfluorocarbon (PFC) liquid is a dense, clear synthetic liquid used as an intraoperative adjunct during vitrectomy to assist in the repair of complex retinal detachments. PFC liquid can inadvertently migrate into the subretinal space, which is often only identified postoperatively. The risk may be higher with newer small gauge vitrectomy systems.

Clinical Features: Subretinal PFC liquid appears as a localized spherical elevation of the retina (Fig. 12.5.1). The location of the subretinal PFC depends on how the PFC made its way under the retina intraoperatively. If the macula is involved, central visual acuity can be adversely affected.

OCT Features: OCT through a subretinal PFC liquid droplet reveals a **hyporeflective cavity** similar in density to the vitreous space (Fig. 12.5.2). The overlying retina is thin due to a mechanical effect of the dense liquid. Sometimes, it can appear as if the PFC liquid is within the retina, though it is actually underneath (Fig. 12.5.3).

Ancillary Testing: None.

Treatment: If the PFC liquid is under the macula and affecting visual acuity, it can be removed. This requires performing a vitrectomy and using a small gauge cannula (41 G) to create an access retinotomy for direct drainage.

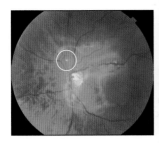

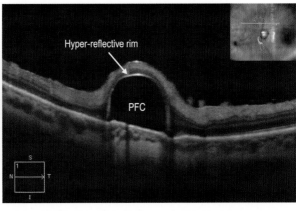

Figure 12.5.1 Color photograph of a retained subretinal PFC liquid droplet superonasal to the optic nerve (circle) following repair of a complex retinal detachment with a giant retinal tear and silicone oil tamponade. *(Courtesy of Caroline Baumal, MD.).*

Figure 12.5.2 OCT through the subretinal PFC liquid droplet (corresponding to Figure 12.5.1) shows a completely hyporeflective space occupied by the PFC. There is a distinct rim of hyper-reflectivity. The overlying retina is very thin due to a mechanical effect of the dense liquid. *(Courtesy of Caroline Baumal, MD.).*

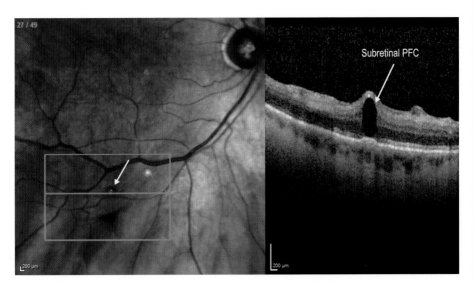

Figure 12.5.3 OCT through a small, retained subretinal PFC liquid droplet (arrows). The PFC appears to be within the retina although it is actually underneath the retina. *(Courtesy of Jeffrey S. Heier, MD.)*

12.6 | X-Linked Juvenile Retinoschisis

Introduction: X-Linked juvenile retinoschisis (XLRS) is the most common type of child-onset retinal degeneration in males and is caused by a mutation in the *RS1* gene.

Clinical Features: There is almost always schisis in the fovea, which is often accompanied by schisis in the peripheral retina (50% of affected eyes), usually inferotemporally. The foveal schisis leads to a characteristic clinical appearance similar to cystoid macular edema with a radial spoke-like pattern (Fig. 12.6.1).

OCT Features: There is **splitting within different retinal layers** involving both the **inner** and **outer** retina. Within the macula, the **inner nuclear layer** is most commonly affected layer (Fig. 12.6.2), though the outer nuclear layer, ganglion cell layer, and nerve fiber layer can all be affected (Fig. 12.6.3). Unlike typical CME the splitting can occur well outside the foveal area.

Ancillary Testing: Fluorescein angiography can be helpful in distinguishing this condition from CME due to other diseases. In XLRS, there is no macular leakage on FA. ERG testing shows a negative waveform. Genetic testing is confirmatory.

Treatment: There is no specific treatment for the disease, but treatment of retinal complications such as retinal detachment may be required.

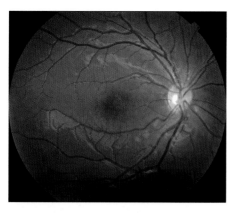

Figure 12.6.1 Color photograph of XLRS shows cystoid changes within the fovea arranged in a characteristic radial spoke-like pattern.

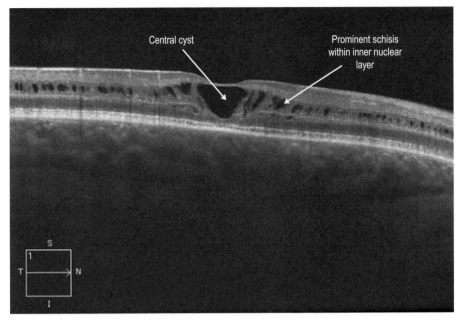

Figure 12.6.2 OCT shows prominent schisis mostly within the inner nuclear layer. There is a central cyst present.

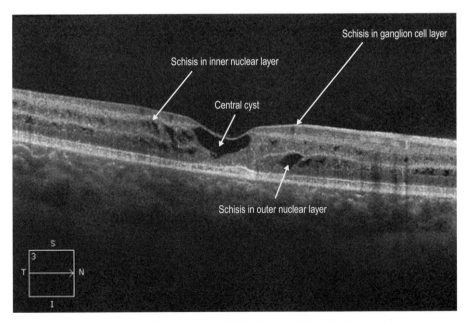

Figure 12.6.3 OCT (corresponding to Figure 12.6.1) shows schisis within the ganglion cell layer, inner nuclear layer, and outer nuclear layer. There is also a central cyst present.

PART 4: Retinal Vascular Disorders

Introduction: Diabetic retinopathy (DR) is the most common cause of new onset blindness in people between the ages of 20 and 74 years in developed countries. DR is estimated to eventually affect one-third of patients with diabetes. The prevalence and severity are affected by the duration of diabetes, glycemic control, and the presence of concurrent hypertension. It is estimated that in 2005–2008, 4.2 million (28.5%) people with diabetes aged 40 years or older had DR, and of these, almost 0.7 million (4.4% of those with diabetes) had advanced DR

Clinical Features: In the early stages, non-proliferative diabetic retinopathy (NPDR) is typically asymptomatic. Retinal manifestations of DR are caused by a microangiopathy that manifests itself as microaneurysms; the hallmarks of NPDR are intraretinal hemorrhages, cotton wool spots, hard exudates, and, in some eyes, macular edema (Fig. 13.1.1). Venous beading and intraretinal microvascular abnormalities may happen in severe NPDR. NPDR is sub-classified as mild, moderate or severe based on the presence and severity of these findings.

OCT Features: Although OCT scanning is not needed for the diagnosis of any form of DR, OCT findings of DR are well characterized on OCT. However, small intraretinal hemorrhages seen in the early stages of diabetes may not be detectable on even high resolution line scans. Microaneurysms appear as **hyper-reflective foci**, mostly within the outer half of the retina, usually spanning more than one retinal layer. They typically have an **inner homogenous lumen** with moderate reflectivity surrounded by a **hyper-reflective** rim. Hyporeflectivity around the microaneurysm is usually associated with leakage on fluorescein angiography. Microaneurysm closure may be associated with resolution of hyper-reflectivity or by a smaller lumen with heterogenous hyper-reflectivity (Figs 13.1.2 to 13.1.4).

Cotton wool spots appear as areas of moderate hyper-reflectivity within the nerve fiber layer. Larger cotton wool spots show shadowing. Hard exudates are also seen as small, relatively well demarcated hyper-reflective clusters usually deeper within the retina and may span multiple layers. Another OCT parameter seen in diabetic patients is presence of hyper-reflective foci within the outer retina on OCT scanning, especially in diabetic macular edema (Fig. 13.1.2). These hyper-reflective foci probably represent a variety of microstructural pathologies including microaneurysms and hard exudates. The baseline amount of hyper-reflective foci seems to correlate positively with HbA1c values.

Diabetic macular edema (DME) is the primary cause of visual loss in NPDR. It is covered in chapter 13.2.

Ancillary Testing: Fluorescein angiography in NPDR is invaluable in looking for microaneurysms, areas of macular and peripheral ischemia and neovascularization. Red free photographs may enhance visualization of the microaneurysms.

Treatment: Glycemic control and management of co-morbidities such as blood lipid levels and hypertension are the mainstays of management of NPDR.

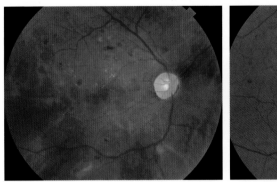
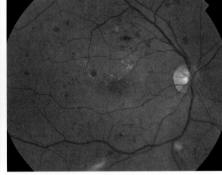

Figure 13.1.1 Color fundus photograph showing intraretinal hemorrhages, microaneurysms, cotton wool spots and hard exudates in a patient with NPDR. The red free photo is especially useful in evaluating for microaneurysms.

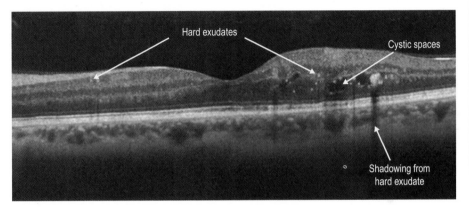

Figure 13.1.2 OCT line scan in a diabetic shows hyper-reflective clusters most likely representing hard exudates between the inner plexiform and the inner nuclear layer.

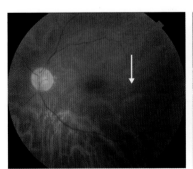
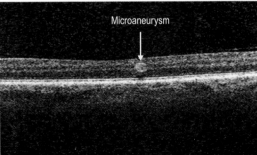

Figure 13.1.3 Photo and OCT line scan through a microaneurysm (white line) showing a discrete, well demarcated area of hyper-reflectivity characteristic of diabetic microaneurysms.

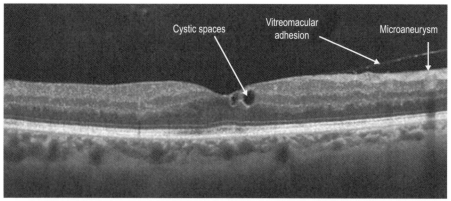

Cystic spaces

Vitreomacular adhesion

Microaneurysm

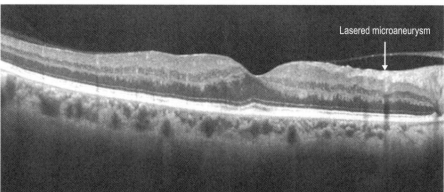

Lasered microaneurysm

Figure 13.1.4 The upper image is a line scan through a microaneurysm showing an inner retinal discrete microaneurysm spanning several layers with a hyper-reflective border and relatively hypo-reflective lumen (arrow). The image below shows a post-focal laser OCT line scan through the same microaneurysm showing shrinkage and hyper-reflectivity throughout the now occluded lumen.

13.2 | Diabetic Macular Edema

Introduction: Diabetic retinopathy is estimated to affect one-third of people with diabetes. The prevalence and severity are affected by the duration of diabetes, glycemic control, and the presence of concurrent hypertension. DME can affect up to 7% of patients with diabetes and is the most common cause of moderate visual loss in diabetic patients.

Clinical Features: The classic clinical descriptions of DME includes focal, diffuse and cystoid (CME), based on the clinical and angiographic appearance (Fig. 13.2.1). Focal macular edema is characterized by focal leaking microaneurysms giving a well-circumscribed area of thickening often associated with hard exudates. Diffuse macular edema is characterized by more widespread vascular abnormalities giving larger areas of thickening, a paucity of hard exudates and cystic changes in the retina. CME associated with DME appears similar to CME from other causes. It is not unusual for affected eyes to manifest two or all three of these sub-types.

OCT Features (Figs 13.2.2 and 13.2.3): In clinical practice as well as in studies, OCT is being used on a routine basis in the diagnosis of DME. Moreover, it is the single most important ancillary test in the management of DME. It is helpful for confirming the clinical diagnosis, choosing the initial therapy and monitoring the edema on follow up or after treatment. Quantitative changes in the OCT in DME are important in following the progression as well as the response to therapy. The mean **central subfield thickness** in the macular map is most often used. More than the absolute number, however, following the evolution of the thickness as well as the 'spread' of the area of thickness is important in the evaluation and follow-up of DME.

The OCT appearance of DME can be categorized into four major types:

▸ Thickening of the fovea with **homogenous optical reflectivity** throughout the whole layer of the retina.
▸ Thickening of the fovea with markedly **decreased optical reflectivity** in mostly the outer retinal layers (cystoid changes).
▸ Thickening of the fovea with **subfoveal fluid** accumulation and distinct outer border of **detached retina**.
▸ Thickening of the fovea with **epiretinal membrane** formation with or without apparent **vitreo-foveal traction**.

The qualitative assessment of OCT scans in DME are proving increasingly important in predicting outcome as well as determining which patients will respond best to individualized treatment. Moreover, OCT may also show foveal microstructural changes such as **disruption of the IS–OS/ ellipsoid layer and of the external limiting membrane**, which may be correlated to visual acuity in DME. Presence of **hyper-reflective foci** may also be associated with severity of the edema in DME and may reduce significantly with successful treatment of edema.

Ancillary Testing: Fluorescein angiography will show microaneurysms in the early and intermediate stages with leakage later on in DME. FA can also be used to evaluate for macular ischemia. Wide field angiography can be used to evaluate for peripheral ischemia and retinal neovascularization.

Treatment: Treatment for DME includes anti-vascular endothelial growth factor therapy, focal or grid laser photocoagulation, intravitreal steroids, and vitrectomy surgery.

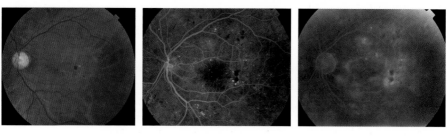

Figure 13.2.1 Fundus photograph of a diabetic patient shows numerous microaneurysms, hard exudates and scattered cotton wool spots. Early frame fluorescein highlights the microaneurysms and late phase shows diffuse leakage at the macula

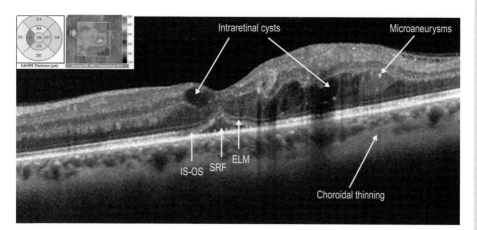

Figure 13.2.2 OCT scanning through the retina shows thickening with outer retinal cystic changes (arrows). The area and extent of thickening can be followed by the false color rendering of the thickness map over the C-scan (inset). The retinal thickness map also provides quantitative information about thickening and is useful in gauging effect of treatment. Also note the hyper-reflective clusters in the outer retina, the trace subretinal fluid or SRF (arrow) and that the external limiting membrane is relatively well-preserved in this patient (arrow) while the IS–OS/ellipsoid layer shows some disruption centrally (arrow).

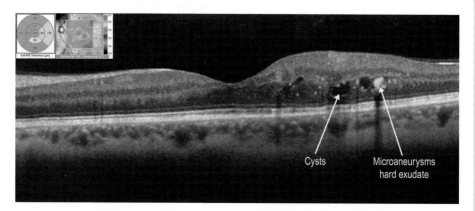

Figure 13.2.3 OCT scan of the same patient after focal laser therapy. The edema and cysts are reduced, as is the retinal thickness on the thickness map. Also, the normal architecture of the IS–OS ellipsoid layer seems relatively well restored.

13.3 | Proliferative Diabetic Retinopathy

Introduction: Proliferative diabetic retinopathy (PDR) is characterized by pathologic retinal neo-vascularization. It can arise from the optic disc (NVD), retina (NVE) and/or the iris (NVI).

Clinical Features: Retinal neovascularization is a hallmark of PDR, which can be seen at the slit lamp as fine networks of blood vessels extending from the retina into the vitreous cavity (Fig. 13.3.1). These vessels can cause visual loss secondary to vitreous hemorrhage, and can induce preretinal fibrosis leading to tractional retinal detachment, retinoschisis, macular edema and combined traction/rhegmatogenous RD

Neovascularization may occur at the disc or elsewhere (NVE) in the retina. It may be preceded by intraretinal microvascular abnormalities (IRMA), which represent a severe form of NPDR.

OCT Features: The typical findings of NPDR are seen in PDR as well. In addition, NVD and NVE may manifest as **loops of hyper-reflective blood vessels** projecting from the retina into the vitre-ous, either at the disc or elsewhere (Fig. 13.3.2). In contrast, areas of IRMA are seen as **disorganization** of the inner retinal vascular architecture with occasional projection beyond the internal limiting membrane, but with no disruption of the hyaloid face (Fig. 13.3.3). The hyaloid may be **thickened** in these cases. In some cases with NVD or NVE, **traction of the retina** with or without retinal detachment may be seen (Fig. 13.3.4).

Ancillary Testing: Fluorescein angiography is the most useful ancillary test in diagnosing diabetic retinopathy. FA of the areas of neovascularization shows profuse dye leakage. Ischemic areas may also be delineated on the FA.

Treatment: PDR is treated with pan-retinal photocoagulation. As it has become clear that elevated levels of VEGF is a critical driver of neovascularization in PDR, increasingly, anti-VEGF therapy is being used as an adjunct in the treatment. There are reports that anti-VEGF injections may induce regression of PDR, but they can cause increased fibrosis of the regressing neovascularization possibly resulting in increased traction on the retina. Vitrectomy is the mainstay of therapy for non-clearing vitreous hemorrhage and traction-related complications of PDR, when pan-retinal photocoagulation fails or is not possible to perform.

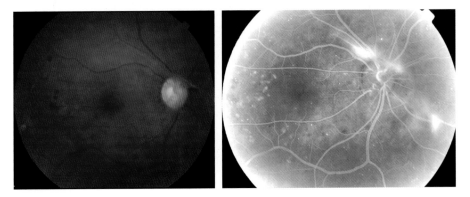

Figure 13.3.1 Neovascularization of the optic disc and of the retina is seen both on the photograph and the accompanying FA.

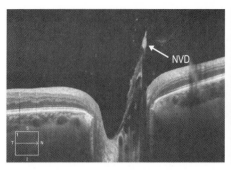
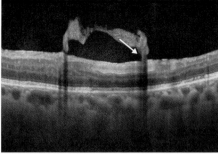

Figure 13.3.2 OCT section through the area of the neovascularization of the optic disc reveals hyper-reflective neovascularization into the vitreous cavity (arrow). The adjacent picture shows a high resolution OCT scan through an area of NVE.

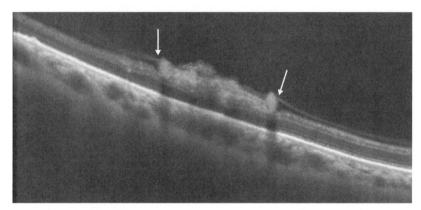

Figure 13.3.3 IRMA/early neovascularization, starting to project into the hyaloid cavity but with an intact, thickened posterior hyaloid face over it (arrows).

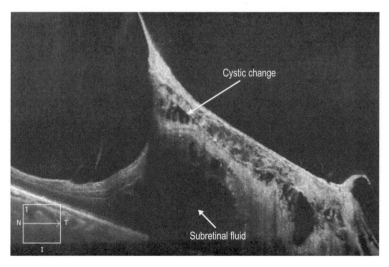

Figure 13.3.4 Tractional retinal detachment. There is thickened preretinal fibrosis and a tractional detachment.

14.1 | Branch Retinal Vein Occlusion

Introduction: Branch retinal vein occlusion (BRVO) is characterized by retinal hemorrhages in the territory of the obstructed vein. Macular edema, retinal ischemia and neovascularization can result, producing visual reduction.

Epidemiology: BRVO usually occurs in patients in their fifth or sixth decades of life. The prevalence of BRVO in developed countries is estimated at just below 1%. There does not appear to be any racial or ethnic predilection. Systemic arterial hypertension is the most common systemic risk factor, present in about 75% of affected patients. The pathogenesis is believed to be disease of the adjacent arterial wall leading to venous compressesion at an arterovenous crossing point.

Clinical Features: Patients may complain of visual blurring, distortion or metamorphopsia. On examination, intraretinal flame and blot shaped hemorrhages as seen in the territory of a dilated, tortuous retinal vein are present (Fig. 14.1.1). Given the distribution of retinal veins the accompanying pathology of BRVO almost never crosses the horizontal raphe. Cotton wool spots, retinal edema in the area drained by the occluded branch, collateral vessels and occasionally retinal neovascularization and vitreous hemorrhage may be seen. Vision loss is largely due to of retinal edema and may sometimes be secondary to retinal ischemia.

OCT Features: OCT shows **retinal thickening and edema** limited to the retinal area drained by the obstructed vein (Figs 14.1.2 and 14.1.3). Macular thickness scans will show retinal thickening, usually confined to half the macula. Line scans through the macula show diffuse retinal edema and **cystic (hyporeflective) spaces** in the outer retina. **Subretinal fluid** may also be observed in severe cases. **Hard exudates** can be seen as small **hyper-reflective intraretinal spots**. Macular thickness scans are particularly valuable in monitoring edema over time and assessing the effects of treatment.

Ancillary Testing: Fluorescein angiography is of value when the hemorrhages start clearing to assess perfusion. It may also be employed earlier to check for retinal neovascularization.

Treatment: Primary treatment of macular edema in a BRVO is intravitreal anti-vascular endothelial growth factor injections. Both intravitreal corticosteroids and grid laser can also be employed, but are second-line therapies. Sector panretinal photocoagulation to reduce the risk of vitreous hemorrhage in the setting of retinal neovascularization is effective.

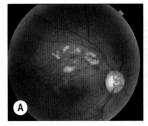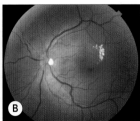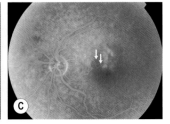

Figure 14.1.1 (A,B) BRVO with a range of findings. Note hemorrhages along the blocked blood vessels, and the cotton wool spots (A) as well as the hard exudates (B). (C) A late frame fluorescein angiogram with collaterals (arrows) and leakage from the vessels.

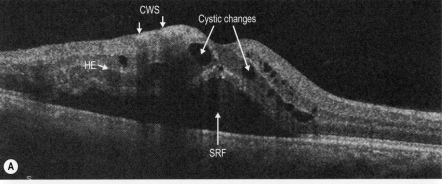

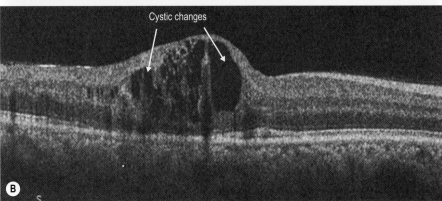

Figure 14.1.2 OCT scans through the macula of the patient (A) with diffuse retinal thickening and cystic changes (arrows). Note the cotton wool spots (CWS) (arrows) in the nerve fiber layer that cause shadowing of the layers beneath them. Some hard exudates (HE) are noted (arrow) as hyper-reflective clusters deeper within the retina and spanning several layers. SRF is also seen (arrow). (B) Note that only part of the retina is thickened unlike in CRVO.

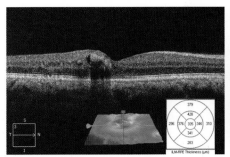

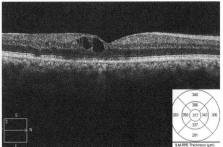

Figure 14.1.3 Successive OCT scans in the same patient after treatment with laser and anti-vascular endothelial growth factor therapy, with thinning of the retina seen on the line and macular thickness scans as well as a smaller geographic spread of the thickening seen on the retinal pigment membrane–internal limiting membrane overlay.

Introduction: Central retinal vein occlusion (CRVO) is due to an obstruction of the central retinal vein at or proximal to the lamina cribrosa. The incidence of CRVO in the US is 30,000 per annum. Risk factors include age >55 years, a history of glaucoma, systemic hypertension, smoking, hyperlipidemia, diabetes, atherosclerosis, coagulopathies, vasculitis, and oral contraceptive use.

Clinical Features: Dilated, tortuous retinal veins and intraretinal hemorrhages are noted in all four quadrants (Fig. 14.2.1). Cotton wool spots, disc edema and macular edema may also be seen. CRVO may be subdivided into ischemic or non-ischemic based on the degree of peripheral retinal non-perfusion seen on fluorescein angiography. Ischemic CRVO tend to have worse visual acuity (<20/200) and more confluent hemorrhage and cotton wool spots. Non-ischemic CRVO usually presents with better visual acuity and the relative paucity of cotton wool spots. Non-ischemic CRVO will convert to ischemic CRVO over weeks to months in about 20–30% of cases. Although the diagnosis of CRVO can be made by the characteristic fundus appearance, perfusion and the presence of ischemia is best assessed by a fluorescein angiogram.

OCT Features: **Macular edema**, a critical feature of CRVO, is best evaluated by an OCT scan (Figs 14.2.2 and 14.2.3). A line scan through the macula shows **diffuse thickening with hyperreflective spaces** within the outer retinal layers consistent with **cystoid macular edema**. Some **subretinal fluid** may also be noted, which most likely is secondary to excess intraretinal fluid 'overflowing' into the subretinal space.

A macular cube scan shows **diffuse thickening**. Central subfield thickness on a cube scan as well as the topography of the edema on the macular map is an effective way of monitoring macular edema over serial visits as well as response to treatment and correlates well to visual acuity in non-ischemic CRVO.

Ancillary Testing: Intravenous fluorescein angiography may show areas of blocked fluorescence from the intraretinal blood, staining of the vessel walls, a delayed arteriovenous phase, non-perfused areas and perifoveal leakage. In the early stages, the presence of hemorrhage may block fluorescence and make it difficult to assess for ischemia. Moreover, the fluorescein angiogram may not show the full extent of perifoveal leakage because of lack of intact perifoveal vessels. Neovascularization of the retina in CRVO will show diffuse leakage from abnormal blood vessels.

Treatment: There is no known effective mechanism to treat macular ischemia in CRVO. However, macular edema may effectively be treated with intravitreal anti-VEGF agents such as bevacizumab, ranibizumab and aflibercept, as well as intravitreal triamcinolone and a sustained release fluocinolone steroid implant. Neovascularization in CRVO is treated with pan retinal photocoagulation laser. Anti-VEGF agents may also be used as adjuncts in the treatment of neovascularization secondary to CRVO.

FIGURE LEGENDS

Figure 14.2.1 Fundus photograph of a CRVO shows four quadrants of intraretinal hemorrhages, cotton wool spots and retinal edema. The fluorescein angiogram highlights the dilated, tortuous vessels. There is blockage noted because of the intraretinal hemorrhages.

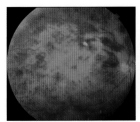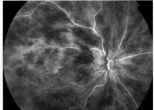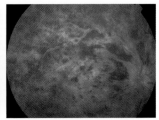

Figure 14.2.1

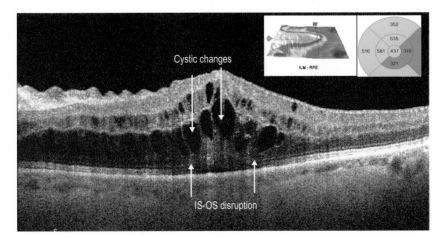

Figure 14.2.2 Intraretinal thickening is noted. Cystic changes are seen in the outer retina that span multiple retinal layers. There is some subretinal fluid. The thickening does not respect the horizontal raphe as seen on the thickness map (inset). There is ellipsoid IS-OS disruption seen.

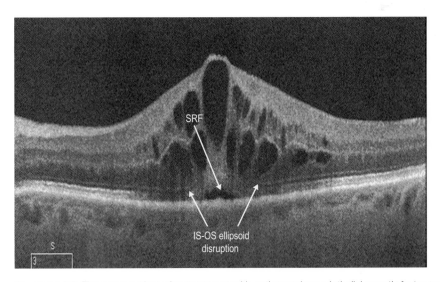

Figure 14.2.3 The same patient after treatment with anti-vascular endothelial growth factor agent. Note that the area of thickening has decreased. There is IS–OS ellipsoid disruption seen and subretinal fluid.

15.1 | Branch Retinal Artery Occlusion

Introduction: The incidence of branch retinal artery occlusion (BRAO) is slightly less than that of central retinal artery occlusion (CRAO), possibly slightly less frequent. Patients typically present with acute painless, monocular vision loss affecting a sector of the visual field. The most common cause is embolus in about two-thirds of cases.

Clinical Features: Retinal whitening is seen along the sector of retina that is supplied by the arterial branch from the central retinal artery (Fig. 15.1.1). The temporal hemisphere is most commonly affected. Emboli are often visualized at the site of blockage, which tends to be at a bifurcation point.

OCT Features: In the acute setting, there is **intense hyper-reflectivity of the inner retinal layers**, similar to that seen in CRAO (see Chapter 15.2), but limited to the sector of retina involved. Vertical, instead of horizontal, OCT cuts can help to make this distinction (Fig. 15.1.2). With time, the edema resolves leaving attenuation and atrophy of the inner retinal layers, which can appear as thinning or even schisis-like changes (Fig. 15.1.3).

Ancillary Testing: Fluorescein angiography can help in securing the diagnosis by revealing a sectoral perfusion deficiency in the acute setting (Fig. 15.1.4).

Treatment: No consistent treatment has demonstrated proven efficacy. Successful YAG laser embolectomy has been described in a few case reports.

FIGURE LEGENDS

Figure 15.1.1 Color fundus photograph shows sectoral retinal whitening (arrowheads) in the distribution of the occluded branch retinal artery. There is also a visible embolus (arrow).

Figure 15.1.2 Acute branch retinal artery occlusion. OCT vertical cut shows inner retinal hyper-reflectivity and thickening only in the sectoral area of retina that is affected by the branch arterial occlusion (left of arrowheads). As with the case in central retinal artery occlusion, the inner hyper-reflectivity in the affected region causes shadowing of the outer layers, which attenuates the signal from the outer retina and retinal pigment epithelium (RPE).

Figure 15.1.3 Inner retinal atrophy with schisis-like changes. Old branch retinal artery occlusion. OCT vertical cut shows inner retinal atrophy with schisis-like changes in the region affected by a branch retinal artery occlusion seven years previously.

Figure 15.1.4 Fluorescein angiography (corresponding to Figure 15.1.1) shows a significant perfusion delay in the sector of retina affected by the branch arterial occlusion.

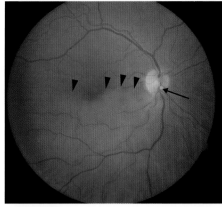

Figure 15.1.1

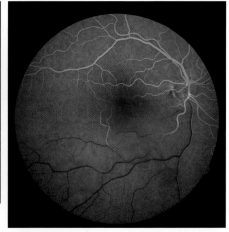

Figure 15.1.4

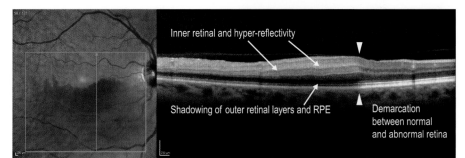

Inner retinal and hyper-reflectivity

Shadowing of outer retinal layers and RPE

Demarcation between normal and abnormal retina

Figure 15.1.2

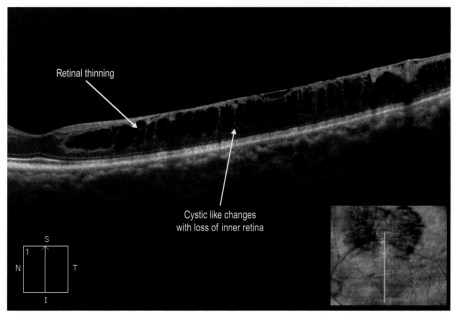

Retinal thinning

Cystic like changes with loss of inner retina

Figure 15.1.3

15.2 Central Retinal Artery Occlusion

Introduction: Central retinal artery occlusion has an incidence of approximately 1 in 10,000 and typically occurs in the seventh decade, affecting men more frequently than woman. Patients present with sudden, profound, painless, monocular vision loss.

Clinical Features: The classic finding is retinal whitening with a central cherry-red spot in the acute setting (Fig. 15.2.1). This corresponds to edema of the inner retina, which is most pronounced in the macula due to the prominent nerve fiber and ganglion cell layer. The central fovea lacks inner retina layers and therefore the underlying retinal pigment epithelium and choroidal pigment shows through giving the cherry-red spot.

OCT Features: In the **acute** setting, there is **intense hyper-reflectivity of the inner retinal layers** (Fig. 15.2.2), corresponding to edema of the retinal layers supplied by the inner retinal vascular supply from the central retinal artery (watershed zone is between inner nuclear and outer plexiform layers). This hyper-reflectivity creates a **shadowing effect, which degrades the normal signal from the outer retinal layers,** therefore providing exaggerated contrast between them. **Later,** the edema resolves leaving **attenuation and atrophy** of the inner retinal layers (see branch retinal artery occlusion case, Chapter 15.1).

Ancillary Testing: Fluorescein angiography is helpful in assessing the perfusion status of the retina and can confirm the diagnosis of CRAO in the acute or subacute setting (Fig. 15.2.3), when suspected on clinical grounds.

Treatment: Though numerous therapies have been attempted, with occasional case reports documenting improvement, none have proven clinical efficacy compared to the natural history.

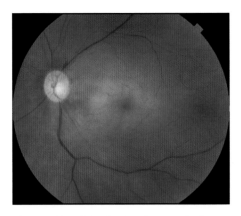

Figure 15.2.1 Color fundus photograph shows a classic cherry-red spot. There is also a superior optic disc hemorrhage.

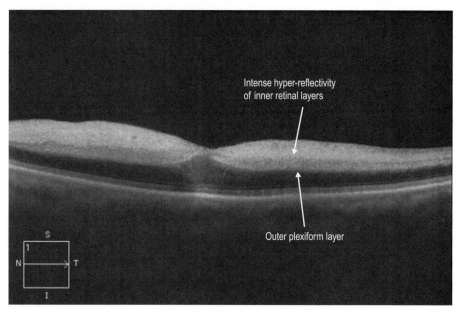

Intense hyper-reflectivity
of inner retinal layers

Outer plexiform layer

Figure 15.2.2 OCT shows fairly homogeneous hyper-reflectivity and thickening of the inner retinal layers with a sharp demarcation at the level of the outer plexiform layer. The hyporeflectivity of the outer retinal layers is exaggerated by a shadowing effect due to the overlying edema.

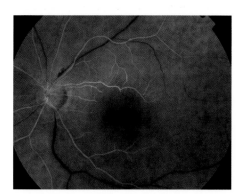

Figure 15.2.3 Fluorescein angiography in the subacute setting of a central retinal artery occlusion at 34 seconds, shows a global, severe delay in filling time of both the arterial and venous circulation. There is also severe central macular ischemia.

15.3 | Cilioretinal Artery Occlusion

Introduction: Cilioretinal artery occlusion (CiRAO) represents the rarest type of retinal vascular disease accounting for less than 10% of retinal arterial occlusions. They can occur isolated, in conjunction with a CRVO, or associated with arteritic ischemic optic neuropathy from giant cell arteritis. When isolated, a collagen vascular disorder may be present. Patients typically report an acute, painless central scotoma or decrease in central visual acuity. When isolated or associated with CRVO, they have a generally good prognosis for at least partial visual recovery.

Clinical Features: There is localized retinal whitening due to inner retinal edema corresponding to the distribution of the cilioretinal artery (Fig. 15.3.1), which is only present in 20–30% of individuals.

OCT Features: **Localized inner retinal hyper-reflectivity**, similar to that seen in branch retinal artery occlusion, but localized to the distribution of the cilioretinal artery is seen acutely (Fig. 15.3.2). Later, OCT will show thinning of the retina in the region supplied by the cilioretinal artery, which is best appreciated by a retinal thickness segmentation map (Fig. 15.3.3).

Ancillary Testing: Fluorescein angiography in the acute setting is helpful to confirm the diagnosis. The cilioretinal artery normally fills with the choroidal circulation, a second or two earlier than the retinal circulation, a key distinction from central or branch retinal artery occlusions.

Treatment: No treatment is of proven clinical efficacy. Corticosteroids are indicated to prevent further visual loss in the setting of giant cell arteritis, but rarely improves the vision.

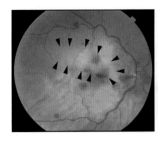

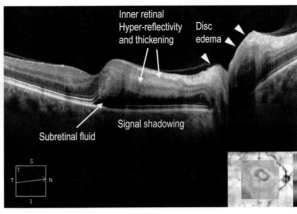

Figure 15.3.1 Color fundus photograph shows localized retinal whitening in the superior macula (arrowheads) corresponding to the distribution of the cilioretinal artery. There are also intraretinal hemorrhages, disc edema, and dilated and tortuous veins due to the concomitant presence of a central retinal vein occlusion.

Figure 15.3.2 OCT (corresponding to Figure 15.3.1) in the acute setting of a CiRAO shows inner retinal hyper-reflectivity and thickening of the inner retinal layers with underlying shadowing. There is a tiny pocket of subretinal fluid. There is also associated disc edema (arrowheads) due to the concomitant CRAO.

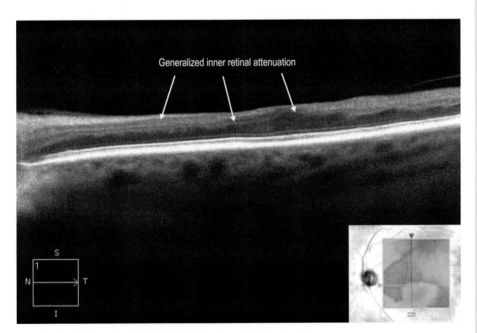

Figure 15.3.3 OCT many years after a cilioretinal artery occlusion shows generalized inner retinal attenuation. Corresponding retinal thickness segmentation map (inset) shows retinal thinning in a region corresponding to the area supplied by the cilioretinal artery.

PART 5: Inherited Retinal Degenerations

16.1 | Retinitis Pigmentosa

Introduction: Retinitis pigmentosa (RP) encompasses a heterogeneous group of inherited disorders that result in loss of retinal cell function (starting with photoreceptors) preferentially in the peripheral retina. Eventually, the macula can be involved in late stages. The prevalence is approximately 1 in 5000. RP can be categorized several different ways: cone–rod versus rod–cone dystrophies, via the inheritence patterns, or by the actual genetic defect, if it is known.

Clinical Features: Nyctalopia is a hallmark feature of the disease. Peripheral vision is impaired early, especially in rod–cone dystrophies, and is slowly progressive. Central vision can also be lost, but typically occurs later in the disease course, although central vision can be impaired at any point by cystoid macular edema. Examination findings include characteristic bone spicule intraretinal deposits, vascular attenuation, and optic nerve pallor (Fig. 16.1.1).

OCT Features: In advanced RP cases, OCT demonstrates marked **attenuation of all retinal layers,** particularly of the **outer retina and photoreceptors** (Fig. 16.1.2). Milder or earlier forms of RP can show more subtle outer retinal atrophy adjacent to a **normal central macula** (Figs 16.1.3 and 16.1.4). OCT can also be helpful to detect the presence of **cystoid macular edema** (Fig. 16.1.5), which is commonly associated with RP.

Ancillary Testing: Electrophysiologic testing, such as multifocal electroretinograms, are helpful to aid in the diagnosis of RP, especially in early cases where clinical findings are mild.

Treatment: There is no widely applicable treatment, but retinal prosthetic implants are now available for very advanced forms of RP.

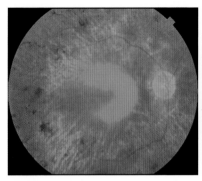

Figure 16.1.1 Color photograph of advanced retinitis pigmentosa shows peripheral bone spicule deposition encroaching into the macula, vascular attenuation, and mild optic nerve pallor.

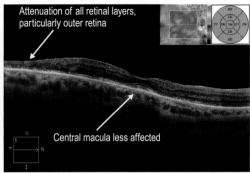

Figure 16.1.2 OCT in advanced retinitis pigmentosa shows significant attenuation of all retinal layers, most notably of the outer retina, and worse temporally. OCT thickness map (inset) shows the degree of generalized retinal thinning throughout the macula. The central macula is affected to a lesser degree than the surrounding area.

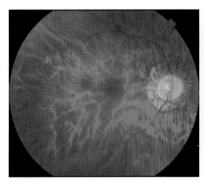

Figure 16.1.3 Color photograph of late onset retinitis pigmentosa with mild disease shows mild pigment deposition and retinal thinning temporal to the macula. There is also unrelated peripapillary atrophy around the optic nerve.

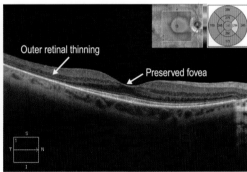

Figure 16.1.4 OCT (corresponding to Figure 16.1.3) shows outer retinal thinning just outside the fovea. OCT thickness map (inset) shows a central island of normal retinal thickness, with significant circumferential thinning outside of this area.

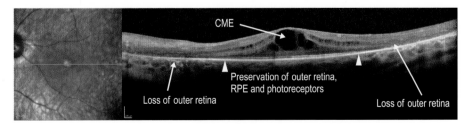

Figure 16.1.5 OCT of a patient with retinitis pigmentosa and associated cystoid macular edema. Despite the CME, the outer retina and photoreceptors are relatively preserved in the central macula (between arrowheads), but are attenuated outside of this area.

16.2 | Stargardt Disease

Introduction: Stargardt disease is the most common inherited macular dystrophy. It is associated with mutations in the *ABCA4* gene and is mostly commonly inherited in an autosomal recessive fashion. The disease has a wide spectrum of severity that accounts for a highly varied presentation.

Clinical Features: There are characteristic 'pisciform' flecks or yellowish deposits that can be in the shape of a fish tail at the level of the RPE. These deposits collect in the posterior pole, usually within the macula, but can be outside the arcades (Fig. 16.2.1). The peripapillary region is characteristically spared. Some cases show severe macular atrophy as the prominent feature.

OCT Features: OCT confirms the **RPE as the location of the abnormal deposits** and shows associated **outer retinal atrophy**, which may be present parafoveally (Fig. 16.2.2) or involve the fovea (Fig. 16.2.3). In more advanced stages of the disease, there is more widespread outer retinal atrophy that can lead to geographic atrophy (Fig. 16.2.4).

Ancillary Testing: Fluorescein angiography and fundus autofluorescence (FAF) can help in confirming the diagnosis. FA can show a characteristic dark choroid (Fig. 16.2.5), present in about 70% of cases. FAF highlights the abnormal RPE deposits and best demonstrates the peripapillary sparing (Figs 16.2.6 and 16.2.7).

Treatment: No treatment is currently available.

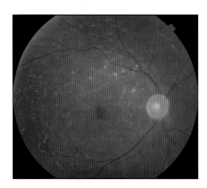

Figure 16.2.1 Color photograph shows numerous pisciform flecks throughout the posterior pole. There are also retinal pigment epithelium abnormalities within the central macula.

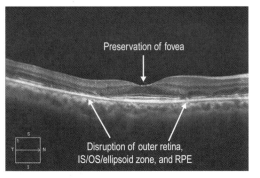

Figure 16.2.2 OCT in a patient with mild Stargardt disease shows a characteristic bulls-eye maculopathy with preservation of the central fovea. There is disruption of the outer retina, IS–OS/ellipsoid zone, and RPE in a parafoveal ring.

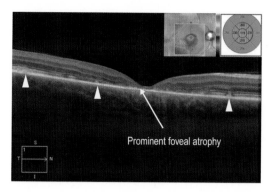

Figure 16.2.3 OCT in a patient with moderate Stargardt disease shows numerous hyper-reflective intra-RPE and/or sub-RPE deposits (arrowheads). There is diffuse loss of the outer retinal layers with prominent foveal atrophy, which is best demonstrated on the OCT thickness map (inset).

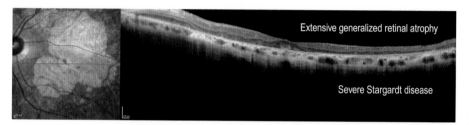

Figure 16.2.4 OCT in a patient with advanced Stargardt disease shows generalized outer retinal atrophy. There is corresponding negative shadowing of the underlying choroidal structures.

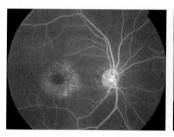

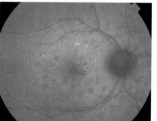

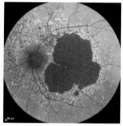

Figure 16.2.5 Mid-phase fluorescein angiography shows staining of central pisciform flecks in addition to a dark choroid.

Figure 16.2.6 FAF corresponding to Figures 16.2.1 and 16.2.2 shows areas of both hyperautofluorescence and hypo-autofluorescence corresponding to pisciform flecks. The characteristic peripapillary sparing is well demonstrated.

Figure 16.2.7 FAF corresponding to Figure 16.2.3 shows areas of both hyperautofluorescence and hypo-autofluorescence corresponding to pisciform flecks. There is a large area of profound central hypo-autofluorescence corresponding to the geographic atrophy. Again, there is characteristic peripapillary sparing.

16.3 | Best Disease

Introduction: Best disease is due to a mutation in the *BEST1* gene and is generally inherited in an autosomal dominant pattern with variable penetrance. *BEST1* mutations are also associated with a variety of other phenotypes, including some cases of adult onset foveomacular dystrophy, autosomal recessive bestrophinopathy, autosomal dominant vitreochoroidopathy, and some cases of rod–cone dystrophy.

Clinical Features: There are multiple clinical phenotypes, which represent different stages of disease and include vitelliform, pseudohypopyon, scrambled egg, and atrophic appearances. The vitelliform stage has an egg yolk appearance of subretinal material, whereas the pseudohypopyon stage exhibits a gravitational layering of the yellow subretinal material with a fluid layer above (Fig. 16.3.1). The disease can be multifocal and asymmetric leading to diagnostic uncertainty. CNV can rarely complicate the course in the atrophic state.

OCT Features: In the vitelliform stage, the **subretinal material** has a **homogeneous**, hyper-reflective appearance. In the pseudohypopyon stage, there is a homogeneous, hyporeflective layer above the hyper-reflective layer (Figs 16.3.2 and 16.3.3) that can be confused with subretinal fluid secondary to CNV. The scrambled egg stage exhibits a mix of retinal pigment epithelium atrophy, pigment clumping, and subretinal fibrosis. The atrophic stage exhibits central atrophy.

Ancillary Testing: Fundus autofluorecence exhibits dramatic hyperautofluorescence (Fig. 16.3.4) and can be very helpful in assisting with the diagnosis. An electro-oculogram typically shows a reduced Arden ratio.

Treatment: No treatment is available except for the secondary CNV that can rarely occur.

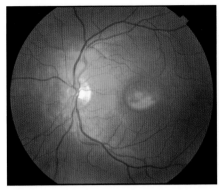

Figure 16.3.1 Color photograph of the pseudohypopyon stage of Best disease.

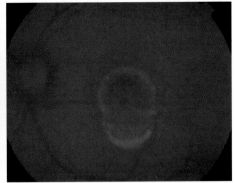

Figure 16.3.4 Fundus autofluorecence exhibits an extremely bright hyperautofluorescence pattern corresponding to lipofuscin deposits in the subretinal space.

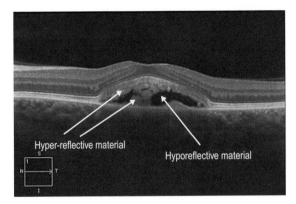

Figure 16.3.2 In the pseudohypopyon stage, a vertical OCT cut in the middle of the lesion would show a hyporeflective top layer (likely to be fluid) and a hyper-reflective bottom layer (likely to be more proteinaceous material) that are sharply demarcated. This example is a horizontal slice, which goes through both layers and shows a mix of both hypo- and hyper-reflective material in the subretinal space.

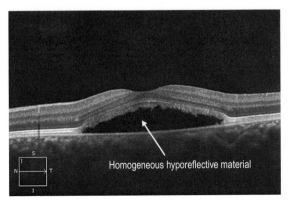

Figure 16.3.3 OCT may show homogeneous hyporeflective material in the subretinal space, which is characteristic of a vitelliform lesion.

16.4 | Cone Dystrophy

Introduction: Cone dystrophy encompasses a heterogeneous group of hereditary retinal dystrophies where isolated cone function is affected primarily.

Clinical Features: The clinical appearance can vary, but a central bulls eye-type maculopathy is most characteristic (Fig. 16.4.1). Early disease may present with a normal clinical examination. Symptoms include loss of visual acuity, color vision, and hemeralopia.

OCT Features: There is initially loss of the **outer retina and photoreceptors** within the **central macula** (Fig. 16.4.2). Over time, this can progress to **complete atrophy**. The peripheral macula and retinal periphery appear normal.

Ancillary Testing: Electrophysiologic testing shows a characteristic pattern where cone function is abnormal, but the rod-isolated scotopic electroretinogram is normal or near normal. This is helpful to differentiate cone dystrophy from cone–rod retinitis pigmentosa.

Treatment: None.

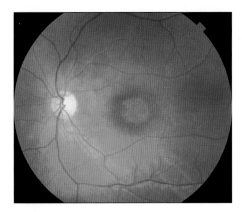

Figure 16.4.1 Color photograph of cone dystrophy shows a central bulls-eye maculopathy.

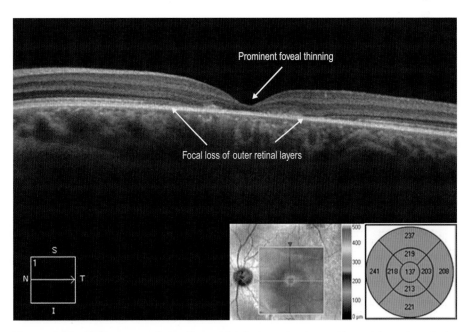

Figure 16.4.2 OCT (corresponding to Figure 16.4.1) shows focal central loss of the outer retinal layers (between arrowheads). There is prominent thinning in the fovea. The corresponding thickness map accentuates the degree of central macular thinning.

111

PART 6: Uveitis and Inflammatory Diseases

17.1 | Multifocal Choroiditis

Introduction: Multifocal choroiditis with panuveitis (MCP) is a common, often idiopathic, usually bilateral, asymmetrical, chronic inflammatory disease occurring predominantly in myopic females in the second to sixth decades of life. Its incidence in the United States is 52.4/100,000 people/years.

Clinical Features: Presentation of MCP is variable. Most patients complain of decreased visual acuity, but photopsia, floaters, blurring of central vision, and enlargement of the blind spot can occur. Anterior segment inflammation may be present but is typically mild. Vitritis of variable severity, and optic disc edema may be present. Multiple small, round to ovoid, pale lesions occur at the level of the outer retina, retinal pigment epithelium (RPE) and choroid, usually 50–350 μm in size, variable in number, and involve mainly the posterior pole (Fig. 17.1.1). Older lesions become pigmented and 'punched-out', resembling histoplasmosis lesions. RPE metaplasia and choroidal neovascularization (peripapillary and macular) are common sequelae. CME, epiretinal membrane and subretinal fibrosis may be seen later.

OCT Features: Active lesions show characteristic **transretinal hyper-reflectivity and drusen-like material** between the RPE and Bruch's membrane (Figs 17.1.2 and 17.1.3). **Nodular collections beneath the RPE** appear to rupture with resulting **inflammatory infiltration** of the subretinal space and the outer retina. Slight **choroidal thickening, localized choroidal hyper-reflectivity** under the lesions, **atrophy of the RPE and the retina** overlying the lesions and **vitreous cells** may be seen. Widespread loss of outer retinal architecture, **retinal thinning**, destructuring of the retinal layers, and **disappearance of IS–OS junction/ellipsoid layer** has also been seen in more advanced cases and may be associated with worse vision. Occasionally, CNV, **CME** and **serous retinal detachments** may be seen

Ancillary Testing: On fluorescein angiography, active lesions show early hypofluorescence due to blockage and late staining (see Fig. 17.1.1). Atrophic lesions show early hyperfluorescence, which fades later, due to RPE window defects. Choroidal neovascularization or CME may be seen in the late phases.

On fundus autofluorescence, macular hyperautofluorescence is seen in areas of active chorioretinitis delineating the diseased area.

On indocyanine green angiography, active lesions show hypofluorescence, and may not be clinically visible. Old lesions show hypofluorescence throughout.

Visual field testing usually reveals an enlarged blind spot, but larger defects may be seen.

Treatment: Topical, periocular and systemic corticosteroid treatment is the mainstay of therapy when the disease is active. Immunosuppressive therapy may be necessary if relentlessly progressive cases. Secondary choroidal neovascularization is not unusual and merits treatment with anti-vascular endothelial growth factor agents, laser photocoagulation, photodynamic therapy, corticosteroids, or a combination thereof.

FIGURE LEGENDS

Figure 17.1.1 Color fundus photograph shows disc edema and hemorrhages and active lesions just nasal to the disc. The lesions are hypofluorescent in the intermediate stages of a fluorescein angiogram.

Figure 17.1.2 OCT through an active choroidal lesion demonstrates 'solid RPE detachments' or drusen-like deposits below the RPE with some overlying RPE and outer retinal atrophy (arrow). Lesions with transretinal hyper-reflectivity are also seen (arrow).

Figure 17.1.3 The OCT scan temporal to the optic nerve shows retinal edema (arrow). Note that the choroid appears thickened and the posterior choroido–scleral border is not visible (arrowhead).

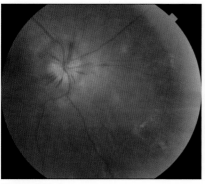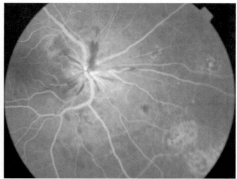

Figure 17.1.1

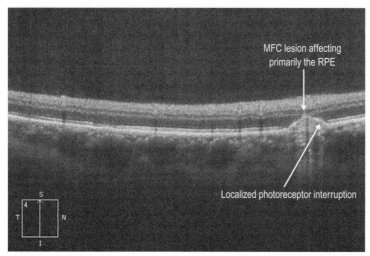

MFC lesion affecting
primarily the RPE

Localized photoreceptor interruption

Figure 17.1.2

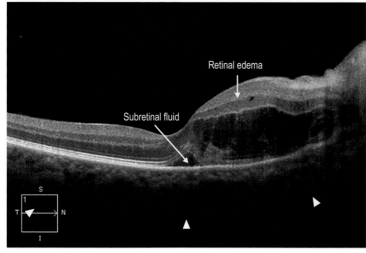

Retinal edema

Subretinal fluid

Figure 17.1.3

17.2 | Birdshot Chorioretinopathy

Introduction: Birdshot retinochoroidopathy, also called vitiliginous chorioretinitis, is a rare bilateral posterior uveitis affecting usually healthy adults between the third to sixth decades of life with a female preponderance. An autoimmune pathogenesis has been suggested with reactivity to the retinal S antigen. There is a strong association with HLA-A29 (>90% of cases). HLA-B44 is also positive in many cases.

Clinical Features: Decreased vision, photopsias, floaters, nyctalopia, and decreased color vision are frequent symptoms. There is minimal to no anterior uveitis with mild vitritis. Multifocal depigmented cream-colored retinal pigment epithelium lesions less than one disc diameter in size are scattered throughout the fundus, although these may be absent or very subtle in the early stages of the disease (Fig. 17.2.1). Retinal phlebitis, narrowing and sheathing of retinal vasculature, disc edema, optic atrophy, cystoid macular edema, choroidal neovascularization and epiretinal membrane may also develop.

OCT Features: Lines scan of the macula may show the typical features of birdshot: **epiretinal membrane formation** and **macular edema** (Fig. 17.2.2). **Subretinal fluid** may be seen in severe cases of macular edema. In chronic cases, the macula is **diffusely thin** and **disruption of the IS–OS segment/ellipsoid layer** with **disorganization of the inner retinal layers** and **retinal pigment epithelium atrophy** may be seen (Fig. 17.2.3). Extramacular and enhanced depth OCT images provide greater information than macular scans, because the choroidal lesions themselves can be scanned. Focal and generalized **loss of the IS–OS junction/ellipsoid layer**, loss of retinal architecture and **outer retinal hyper-reflective foci** overlying the lesions is typical. **Generalized thinning** of the choroid and outer retina, and **hyporeflective suprachoroidal space** are other features.

Ancillary Testing: Diagnosis is based on clinical features. On fluorescein angiography, birdshot lesions may block dye in the early phases, and stain in the late phases. All lesions seen on clinical examination may not be evident on FA. There may be retinal vascular leakage, perifoveal capillary leakage, disc edema, staining and late cystoid macular edema. Occasionally, choroidal neovascularization may be seen at the site of old lesions. Indocyanine green angiography reveals early hypofluorescent spots and possible diffuse late leakage. Many more spots may be seen on indocyanine green angiography than on FA further consolidating the theory that this is primarily a choroidal disease.

Electroretinogram shows depressed rod and cone function with a decreased b-wave amplitude and increased latency of the b-wave compared to the a-wave which is relatively preserved. The b-wave may eventually be extinguished in severe cases. The 30 Hz flicker response is delayed with increased implicit times.

HLA testing (HLA-A29) is positive in 80–96% of patients.

Treatment: The mainstay of treatment is periocular and systemic steroids. Steroid sparing treatments used include cyclosporine, azathioprine, methotrexate, infliximab, immunoglobulins, and mycophenolate mofetil. Targeted treatments are being studied.

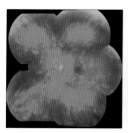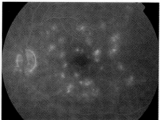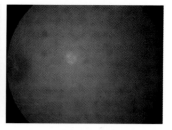

Figure 17.2.1 Characteristic fundus photograph of a patient with birdshot with hypopigmented lesions noted extending into the mid-periphery. Late frames of the fluorescein angiography show hyperfluorescence, and late-frame indocyanine green angiography shows the lesions as hypofluorescent spots with some diffuse hyperfluorescence.

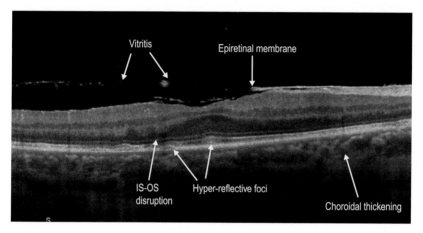

Figure 17.2.2 OCT scan shows vitritis, epiretinal membrane formation and disruption of the IS–OS/ellipsoid layer with some inner retinal disorganization.

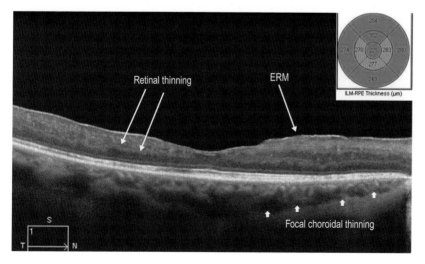

Figure 17.2.3 OCT in late stage birdshot showing thinning of the retina with preferential loss of outer retinal layers.

17.3 | Serpiginous Choroiditis

Introduction: Serpiginous choroiditis, also known as helicoid or geographic choroidopathy, is a rare, idiopathic inflammatory disease affecting the retinal pigment epithelium, outer retina, and the inner choroid. It is slightly more common in men between 30 and 70 years of age with no predilection for race. It usually occurs in otherwise healthy individuals.

Clinical Features: The most common complaints are blurring of vision and central or paracentral scotomata, but occasionally it is diagnosed asymptomatically on routine examination. Anterior segment inflammation is usually mild, and the vitreous may be clear or show minimal inflammation. The disease can be classified on the basis of clinical presentation as:
- Peripapillary
- Macular
- Ampiginous.

Lesions most commonly start in the peripapillary region (Fig. 17.3.1). Active lesions are yellow to grayish with associated overlying retinal edema. These spread in a centripetal, helicoid, map-like or snake-like pattern, from the initial area of involvement. Active lesions become atrophic in weeks to months, with atrophy of the retinal pigment epithelium, choriocapillaris, and choroid. New lesions arise at the edge of the atrophic ones. Choroidal neovascularization, subretinal hemorrhage and serous retinal detachment can complicate the course. The disease is typically chronic and remitting with quiescent periods of up to several years between active episodes.

OCT Features: The characteristic active lesion of serpiginous choroiditis shows **hyper-reflectivity and thickening of the outer retina, and increased reflectance of the choroid**. This has been referred to as the 'waterfall' effect (Fig. 17.3.2). There is also **disruption of the photoreceptor inner and outer segment junction** in both active and inactive lesions (Fig. 17.3.3).

Ancillary Testing: Visual field examination reveals central or paracentral scotoma. Fluorescein angiography of the active lesions show early hypofluorescence and late hyperfluorescence in a typical geographic pattern. Retinal vessels may stain adjacent to the active lesions. Old lesions show window defects, and late staining (see Figs 17.3.1D–F). Indocyanine green angiography reveals choroidal non-perfusion (see Fig. 17.3.1C).

Fundus hyperautofluorescence provides a clear demarcation of the retinal pigment epithelium damage in acute lesions. Scarring of the lesions causes decreased autofluorescence.

Treatment: Periocular and systemic corticosteroids have been used to treat acute episode and long-term steroid-sparing therapy such as cyclosporine, azathioprine, cyclophosphamide, interferon alpha-2a or infliximab are needed to prevent recurrence.

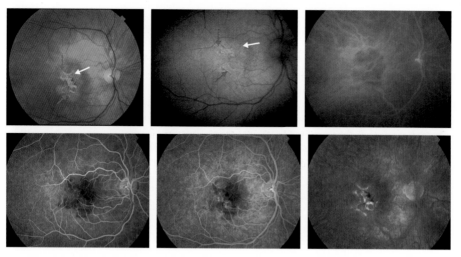

Figure 17.3.1 Color photographs and autofluorescence show macular serpiginous, with old inactive lesion (red arrow) and active lesion at the margin (white arrow). Indocyanine green angiography shows choroidal hypofluorescence consistent with areas of activity. Fluorescein angiography shows early hypofluorescence and late hyperfluorescence.

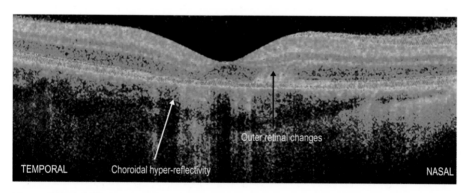

Figure 17.3.2 OCT shows choroidal hyper-reflectivity (white arrow), outer retinal thickening (black arrow) and disruption of the ellipsoid IS–OS layer.

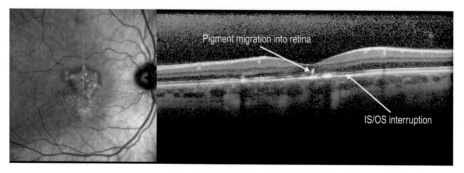

Figure 17.3.3 The same patient in Figure 17.3.2 after treatment with steroids. Note resolution of the choroidal hyper-reflectivity and retinal thickening.

17.4 Vogt–Koyanagi–Harada Disease

Introduction: Vogt–Koyanagi–Harada (VKH) disease is a rare, bilateral, chronic, idiopathic, granulomatous panuveitis. It occurs predominantly in females, usually between 30 and 50 years old, with a propensity for dark pigmented races: Asians, Hispanics, Native Americans and Asian Indians. An immune reaction to uveal melanocytes has been proposed as the mechanism, but the cause largely remains unknown.

Clinical Features: Initially, VKH was classified as two separate diseases:
▸ Vogt–Koyanagi syndrome: comprising chronic anterior uveitis, alopecia, poliosis, vitiligo, and dysacousia.
▸ Harada's disease: comprising bilateral posterior, exudative uveitis, and neurological features.
Considering the considerable overlap in the features, the term VKH disease is now used.

At onset, patients may experience flu-like symptoms, central nervous system signs, optic neuropathy, sensitivity of hair and skin to touch, perilimbal vitiligo, alopecia, vitiligo poliosis and auditory signs. Blurred vision, photophobia, conjunctival hyperemia, and ocular pain also occur. Bilateral anterior and exudative posterior uveitis is typical. Shallow, serous retinal detachments are seen at the posterior pole with underlying choroidal infiltrates (Fig. 17.4.1). The optic disc is edematous and hyperemic.

With resolution of the uveitis and retinal detachments, a gradual depigmented appearance of the choroid (sunset-glow fundus) may develop.

OCT Features: OCT reveals **serous retinal detachments** at the macula. The **subretinal fluid** may reveal a higher optical density than the vitreous, suggesting a higher level of protein content (Figs 17.4.2 and 17.4.3). Inner retinal layers are typically well preserved with **cystic changes** and complex infolding in the outer retinal layers. **Subretinal fibrinoid deposits** are seen, which may later evolve into **subretinal fibrosis**. **Vitreoretinal interface alterations** with cellular deposits may also be seen. There may be alteration and **thickening of the IS–OS junction/ellipsoid layer, RPE and choroidal folds**, and **thickening of the choroid**. Enhanced depth imaging OCT will show significant choroidal thickening, which resolves when treated.

Ancillary Testing: On fluorescein angiography, active disease with subretinal exudation appears as multiple hyperfluorescent dots at the RPE level, which gradually enlarge and coalesce as the dye accumulates in the subretinal space. With resolution of the exudative phase, these features no longer are visualized. The chronic phase is characterized by diffuse scattered hyperfluorescent dots corresponding to window defects at the RPE level.

On fundus autofluorescence, serous detachments are observed to be hypoautofluorescent, due to blockage. Hypoautofluorescent multiple, granular dots are seen after resolution, which correspond to the window defects on FA.

On indocyanine green angiography, active disease is characterized by choroidal stromal vasculature hyperfluorescence and leakage, disc hyperfluorescence, hypofluorescent dots, and indistinct, fuzzy large choroidal vessels with decreased dye filling.
▸ Ultrasonography: Ultrasound is helpful if the posterior segment is not visible, and reveals diffusely thickened posterior choroid with low to medium reflectivity, serous retinal detachments, vitritis, and thickened sclera or episclera.
▸ Cerebrospinal fluid analysis: cerebrospinal fluid pleocytosis and elevated protein levels are seen.

Treatment: Topical, periocular and systemic steroids are instituted as therapy, along with topical cycloplegics. In chronic or non-responsive cases, or when side effects from steroids are severe, other agents are employed including cyclosporine, chlorambucil, cyclophosphamide, azathioprine or infliximab.

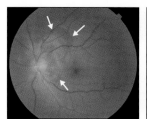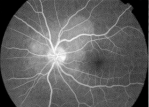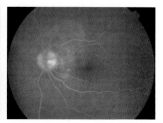

Figure 17.4.1 Color fundus photograph of a patient with Vogt–Koyanagi–Harada shows the classic exudative posterior pole detachment (arrows). Intermediate stage fluorescein angiography shows multiple hyperfluorescent spots at the choroidal level and some diffuse pooling of dye in the subretinal space. Late stage fluorescein angiography shows disc hyperemia and staining with pooling of dye in the serous retinal detachment.

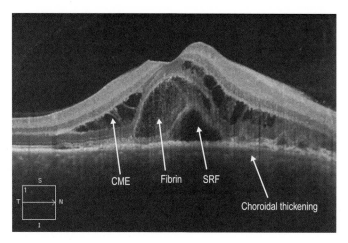

Figure 17.4.2 OCT scan through the macular detachment in a patient with Vogt–Koyanagi–Harada shows the turbid subretinal fluid (SRF) with fibrin deposition. There are outer retinal cystic changes seen. The retina is thickened.

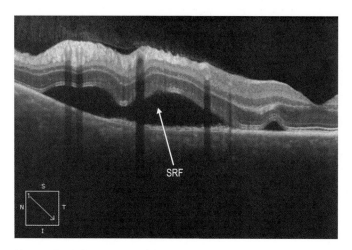

Figure 17.4.3 Extramacular OCT scan shows subretinal fluid. Note that the choroid is thickened and the choroidoscleral border is not visible.

17.5 | Sympathetic Ophthalmia

Introduction: Sympathetic ophthalmia is an exceedingly rare, bilateral diffuse granulomatous uveitis that develops following ocular penetrating trauma or surgery. Inflammation in the contralateral, unaffected eye develops days to years after the event, but usually occurs within three months of the injury.

Epidemiology: Sympathetic ophthalmia is rare, affecting 0.2–0.5% of all traumatic penetrating eye injuries and 0.007% of patients after ocular surgery featuring a penetrating incision. The risk after pars plana vitrectomy is 0.01%.

Clinical Features: Clinically, patients present with a bilateral severe, unremitting granulomatous panuveitis. There may be associated hypotony, small depigmented nodules at the level of the retinal pigment epithelium (Dalen–Fuch's nodules), choroidal thickening, and serous retinal detachments (Fig. 17.5.1). Signs of prior injury or surgery in one eye are present.

OCT Features: OCT findings include **posterior choroidal thickening** and accumulation of **turbid subretinal fluid** with deposition of fibrin and/or fibrinous bands in the subretinal fluid (Fig. 17.5.2). **Macular edema** may also be seen. In later stages of sympathetic ophthalmia, there is retinal and retinal pigment epithelium **atrophy and thinning** with **transmission defects** noted (Fig. 17.5.3).

Treatment: Sympathetic ophthalmia can be prevented by enucleation of a blind, injured eye within two weeks after the trauma. Even after the onset of sympathetic ophthalmia, it may be of help to enucleate the eye that previously obtained injury. Once sympathetic ophthalmia is established in the contralateral eye, the mainstay of treatment consists of systemic anti-inflammatory agents such as oral corticosteroids or other immunosuppressive agents. More recently, treatments with local injections of corticosteroids in combination with or without systemic therapy, and intravitreal injections of infliximab have been reported.

Severe cases of sympathetic ophthalmia may be refractory to treatment.

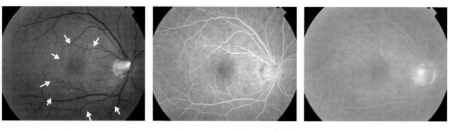

Figure 17.5.1 Red-free photo of a macular serous detachment associated with sympathetic ophthalmia. The fluorescein angiogram shows pooling in the subretinal space associated with a serous retinal detachment.

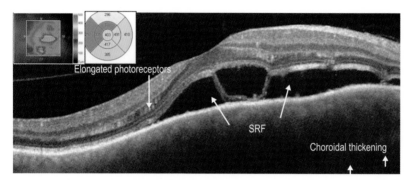

Figure 17.5.2 OCT scan through the macula shows a serous retinal detachment with fibrin deposits and bands (arrows). The choroid is thickened (arrows) and the photoreceptors appear elongated. The thickness map shows thickening in the region with the serous retinal detachment.

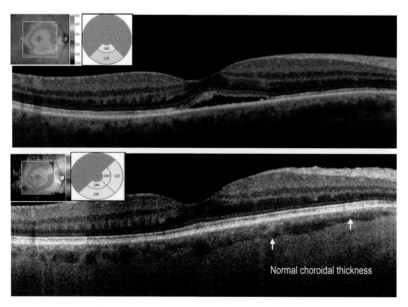

Figure 17.5.3 Sequential post treatment OCTs show resolution of the subretinal fluid and the retinal detachment. Note that the choroidal thickness is reduced (arrows).

17.6 | Posterior Scleritis

Introduction: Posterior scleritis is uncommon inflammation of the sclera occurring posterior to the insertion of the rectus muscles. Posterior scleritis can occur in isolation or in association with anterior scleritis. There is strong female preponderance due it is association with autoimmune disorders. Scleritis has been associated with many systemic diseases, but the strongest association is with rheumatoid arthritis. It usually occurs in the fourth to sixth decades of life. Infectious scleritis has also been reported, but infectious posterior scleritis is rare.

Clinical Features: Common presenting features are pain, tenderness, blurred vision, proptosis and pain or restriction of eye movements. One-third of patients will have no pain. Common findings include retinal striae, exudative retinal detachment and choroidal thickening and detachments (Fig. 17.6.1). Less common manifestations are macular and disc edema, subretinal mass, hemorrhages and exudation. Diagnosis may be difficult in the absence of anterior scleritis.

OCT Features: CME can occur but **serous macular and retinal detachments** are most common. The choroid may be **thickened** on enhanced depth imaging scanning (Figs 17.6.2 and 17.6.3).

Ancillary Testing: Fluorescein angiography is strikingly similar to that seen in Vogt–Koyanagi–Harada disease, with subretinal leakage points which coalesce in the late phases. B-scan ultrasonography reveals fluid in the sub-Tenon's space that may manifest as the classic 'T-sign'. Scleral thickening is also seen. Exudative retinal detachments may also be visualized. Computed tomography or magnetic resonance imaging scan of the orbits may show diffuse thickening of the sclera (the 'ring 360° sign' on computed tomography scanning).

Treatment: Systemic associations should be ruled out. Non-steroidal anti-inflammatory drug therapy, oral corticosteroid therapy, or in recalcitrant or recurrent cases, immunosuppressive drugs are effective treatments.

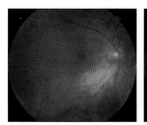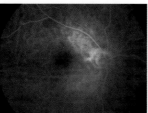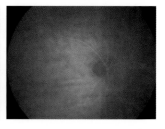

Figure 17.6.1 Fundus photograph of a patient with posterior scleritis showing some obscuration of choroidal detail and subtle choroidal folds better seen on the accompanying fluorescein angiography and indocyanine green angiography.

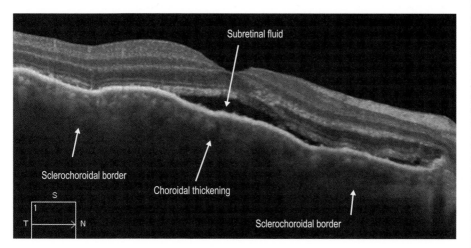

Figure 17.6.2 OCT scanning through the macula reveals a serous macular detachment. There is choroidal thickening seen and the posterior extent of the choroid cannot be visualized on the OCT scan.

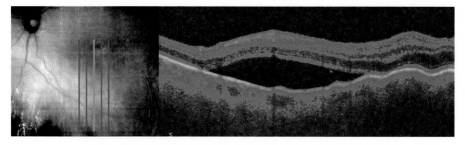

Figure 17.6.3 OCT scan showing relatively flat macula but with gravitation of the exudative retinal detachment inferiorly.

18.1 Toxoplasmic Chorioretinitis

Introduction: Toxoplasmosis is a zoonotic infection caused by the protozoan parasite *Toxoplasma gondii*. It is the most common cause of posterior uveitis and focal retinitis. The disease typically affects immunocompetent individuals.

Clinical Features: In recurrent cases, there is a characteristic focus of active chorioretinitis with overlying vitritis adjacent to a pigmented chorioretinal scar (Fig. 18.1.1). Associated retinal vasculitis may be present. The disease is almost always unilateral. Primary infection may present with a similar appearance in the absence of a pigmented scar (Fig. 18.1.2). Multifocality and bilaterality are rare except in immunocompromised individuals. In elderly patients, a severe form of toxoplasmosis that is relentlessly progressive, resembling acute retinal necrosis, can occur.

OCT Features: Peripheral lesions are often not amenable to imaging with OCT but if located within or near the macula, OCT reveals **thickening and distortion of all the retinal layers** and the retinal pigment epithelium (Fig. 18.1.3) within the area of active chorioretinitis. **Kyrieleis plaques** are a non-specific finding that can be present **overlying retinal blood vessels** in the setting of vasculitis from toxoplasmic chorioretinitis. These appear as hyper-reflective round outpouchings or plaque-like deposits on the surface of both arteries and veins (Fig. 18.1.4). Choroidal neovascularization can occur secondarily from toxoplasmosis scars and OCT can show associated intraretinal and subretinal fluid.

Ancillary Testing: Fluorescein angiography can be helpful, but is not necessary. Clinical examination is typically enough to confirm the diagnosis. If the diagnosis is in doubt, intraocular fluid sampling with polymerase chain reaction testing can be confirmative.

Treatment: The disease course is most frequently self-limited and proof of treatment efficacy is lacking. Disease threatening the macula or optic nerve is more apt to be treated. Numerous strategies of various oral and intravitreal antimicrobial agents have been used.

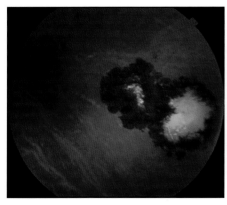

Figure 18.1.1 Color photograph of a typical toxoplasmosis chorioretinal scar with resolving active retinitis.

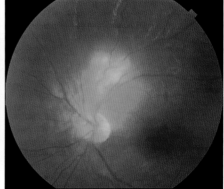

Figure 18.1.2 Color photograph of primary toxoplasmosis chorioretinitis superior to the optic nerve in a 14-year-old female who had congenital toxoplasmosis infection.

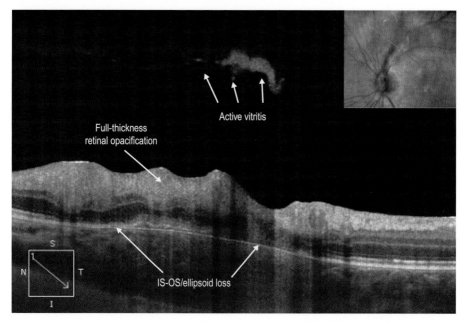

Figure 18.1.3 OCT using enhanced depth imaging protocol (corresponding to Figure 18.1.2) shows distortion and thickening of all retinal layers in the area of active chorioretinitis. The inner retinal layers are more involved and are hyper-reflective. There are patchy areas of IS–OS/ellipsoid zone and retinal pigment epithelium loss. An area of active vitritis is visible.

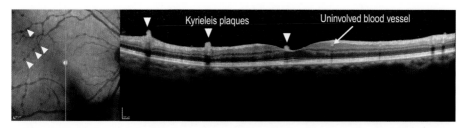

Figure 18.1.4 OCT vertical line scan and corresponding infrared image through Kyrieleis plaques reveals hyper-reflective circular opacities (arrowheads) overlying both retinal arterioles and venules.

18.2 Tuberculosis

Introduction: *Mycobacterium tuberculosis* can infect many extrapulmonary organs, including the eyes. It is a common infectious cause of uveitis in certain, mostly tropical, countries. HIV-infected patients are particularly at risk to disease.

Clinical Features: Ocular manifestations include choroidal granuloma, choroiditis, chorioretinitis, optic nerve infiltration, and uveitis (Figs 18.2.1 and 18.2.2). Choroidal involvement can cause a large plaque in the posterior pole, similar to that seen in serpiginous choroiditis, or can be multifocal in nature. Multiple old, inactive associated chorioretinal scars are suggestive of tuberculosis.

OCT Features: OCT is particularly useful to image tuberculosis involvement of the retina and choroid. Infiltration in the subretinal space and choroid by a homogeneous material of medium to high reflectivity are typical early in the disease course (Fig. 18.2.3). There can be associated subretinal fluid. Resolving chorioretinitis can leave retinal and choroidal atrophy (Fig. 18.2.4).

Ancillary Testing: Tuberculin skin testing, interferon-gamma release assays, and chest radiography can be used to aid in the diagnosis. Referral for a complete medical evaluation is warranted if tuberulosis is suspected.

Treatment: No directed ocular therapy is indicated. There are numerous systemic anti-tubercular therapeutic agents available. Treatment should be coordinated by an infectious disease specialist.

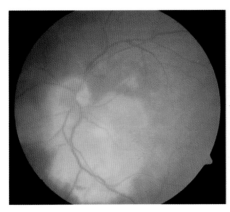

Figure 18.2.1 Color photograph of active tubercular chorioretinitis involving the macula and optic nerve. *(Courtesy of Alay S. Banker, MD.)*

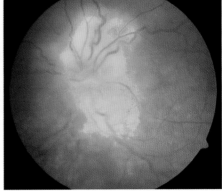

Figure 18.2.2 Color photograph of active tubercular chorioretinitis (superior to optic nerve) and resolving chorioretinitis (in macula). *(Courtesy of Alay S. Banker, MD.)*

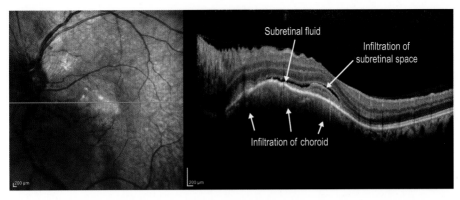

Figure 18.2.3 OCT (corresponding to Figure 18.2.1) shows homogeneous infiltration of the choroid causing an irregular, dome-shaped elevation of the overlying retinal pigment epithelium and retina. There is also infiltration of the subretinal space with a homogeneous material of medium reflectivity and associated subretinal fluid. *(Courtesy of Alay S. Banker, MD.)*

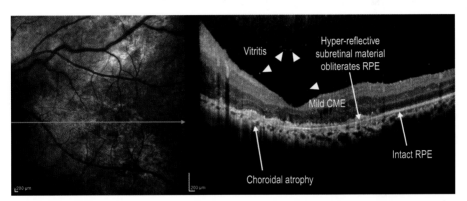

Figure 18.2.4 OCT (corresponding to Figure 18.2.2) of resolving tubercular chorioretinitis shows atrophy of the choroid. The subretinal space has a thin layer of hyper-reflective material that seems to have destroyed the RPE because there is negative shadowing that ends abruptly where the retinal pigment epithelium is intact. Other features include mild CME and small hyper-reflective deposits in the vitreous (arrowheads), which likely represent vitreous infiltration by tuberculosis organisms or secondary inflammation. *(Courtesy of Alay S. Banker, MD.)*

18.3 | Acute Syphilitic Posterior Placoid Chorioretinitis

Introduction: Ocular syphilis is a rare manifestation of disease caused by the spirochete *Treponema pallidum*. Intraocular infection may be acquired during the secondary or tertiary stages of infection. This disease is most prevalent in the fifth decade of life in men. Of note, there is high correlation with co-infection with human immunodeficiency virus type 1.

Clinical Features: Acute syphilitic posterior placoid chorioretinitis is a specific and characteristic manifestation of ocular syphilis. A singular or multiple yellow-colored, circular, deep retinal or choroidal plaques located in the macula are characteristically present. The lesions may be multifocal and subtle. Bilaterality occurs in about half of affected patients.

OCT Features: Much like the disease itself, the OCT findings can vary. Focal loss of the **external limiting membrane** and **IS–OS/ellipsoid zone** are common, the **retinal pigment epithelium layer** may be abnormal, and **choroidal infiltration** with thickening may also be visible (Fig. 18.3.1). Serous retinal detachments involving the macula are uncommon, occurring in about 10% of cases.

Ancillary Testing: Fluorescein angiography usually shows a central hypofluorescent area corresponding to the plaque, occasionally with leopard spotting early, followed by progressive hyperfluorescence later. Late staining from the retinal vessels and optic nerve, even outside areas of retinal whitening, is typical. Indocyanine green angiography typically shows hypofluorescence in both early and late stages.

Treatment: Prompt treatment with intravenous penicillin G (24 million units daily for 14 days) is indicated. Testing should be performed for both human immunodeficiency virus and neurosyphilis.

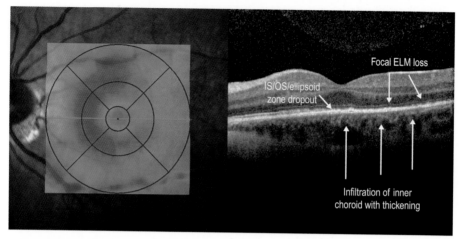

Focal ELM loss

IS/OS/ellipsoid
zone dropout

Infiltration of inner
choroid with thickening

Figure 18.3.1 OCT in acute syphilitic posterior placoid chorioretinitis shows involvement of the IS–OS layer. The IS–OS/ellipsoid zone is abnormally indistinct (between black arrowheads) and then drops out completely (to right of black arrowheads). The retinal pigment epithelium layer in the region of IS–OS/ellipsoid zone dropout is irregular. There is also focal loss of the external limiting membrane and infiltration of the inner choroid with thickening. The accompanying thickness map shows abnormal thickening of the parafoveal region, particularly nasally. *(Courtesy of Robin A. Vora MD.)*

18.4 *Candida Albicans* Endogenous Endophthalmitis

Introduction: *Candida albicans* is the most common pathogen responsible for fungal endophthalmitis. Intravenous drug use, in-dwelling catheters, and immunocompromised host status are risk factors for infection.

Clinical Features: The clinical appearance of *C. albicans* endogenous endophthalmitis is very characteristic. The lesions are typically small areas of chorioretinitis involving the posterior pole, are creamy-white in color and with fairly well-defined borders (Fig. 18.4.1). Overlying vitritis is typical, often in a 'string of pearls' arrangement (Fig. 18.4.2).

OCT Features: *C. albicans* retinal infiltrates are **located superficially** in the retina. They are **hyper-reflective, dome-shaped elevations** overlying the inner retina (Fig. 18.4.3). They obscure the underlying retina due to shadowing. **Signal quality can be poor** due to the presence of overlying inflammatory debris in the vitreous cavity.

Ancillary Testing: Diagnosis is typically made by clinical exam alone. Vitreous biopsy can help confirm the diagnosis.

Treatment: Various antifungal agents are available and can be administered via oral, intravenous, and intravitreal routes dependent on disease severity.

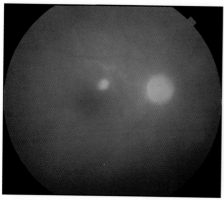

Figure 18.4.1 Color photograph shows a creamy-white, fluffy, well-circumscribed retinal infiltrate in the superonasal macula. There is moderate overlying vitritis.

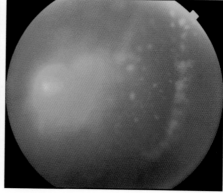

Figure 18.4.2 Color photograph shows many small yellow vitreous opacities connected by inflammatory debris in a characteristic 'string of pearls' arrangement.

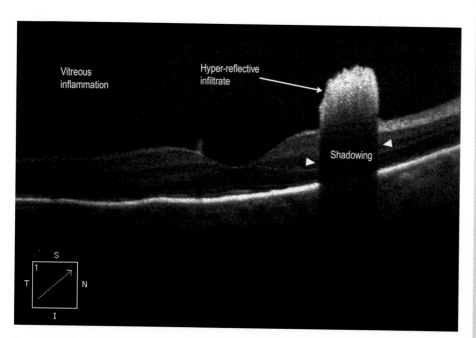

Figure 18.4.3 OCT shows a well-circumscribed, hyper-reflective, dome-shaped elevation overlying the retina (arrow). There is dense shadowing (between arrowheads) obscuring the underlying structures. The overall signal quality of the scan is poor due to moderate vitreous inflammation.

18.5 | Acute Retinal Necrosis Syndrome

Introduction: Acute retinal necrosis (ARN) syndrome, also known as acute herpetic retinitis, is a rare disorder occurring most commonly in immunocompetent adults. The most common etiologic agent is varicella zoster virus, followed by herpes simplex viruses (types 1 and 2).

Clinical Features: ARN commonly presents with multifocal peripheral areas of full-thickness retinal necrosis in well-circumscribed patches that rapidly coalesce in a circumferential pattern (Fig. 18.5.1). There is an associated brisk intraocular inflammatory reaction and an occlusive vasculitis that primarily affects the retinal arteries. Vitritis is universal and a mild anterior chamber reaction with keratic precipitates is typical. Elevated intraocular pressure is not unusual. Without treatment, spread is rapid and may also involve the fellow eye.

OCT Features: In cases where the macula is not directly involved clinically, but is threatened, OCT shows subclinical disease involvement (Fig. 18.5.2), which can be useful for prognostic purposes. Disease activity beyond the clinically evident area of involvement (or leading edge) is typical of this condition. In the setting of frank necrosis involving the macula, OCT reveals **attenuation of all retinal layers**.

Ancillary Testing: Diagnostic sampling of aqueous or vitreous for polymerase chain reaction testing can be very helpful to assist in the diagnosis. Systemic antibody testing rarely is indicated. Serial color wide field photographs can be helpful to monitor disease progression. Fluorescein angiography will show hypofluorescence in the areas of necrosis with a characteristic abrupt cut-off of dye in the blood vessels.

Treatment: Antiviral agents are the mainstay (acyclovir, valacyclovir, valgancyclovir, famcyclovir, foscarnet) and can be delivered orally, intravenously, and intravitreally, or in combination. Vitrectomy is often required after the acute infection is over, for the management of media opacity and retinal detachment, which commonly develop in the healing phase of the disease.

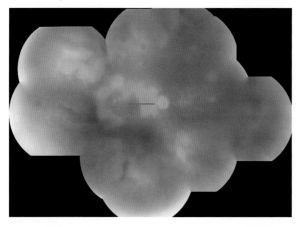

Figure 18.5.1 Color photograph of a patient with acute retinal necrosis at presentation. There is extensive peripheral retinal whitening from necrosis and associated occlusive vasculitis. Red line corresponds to OCT section in next figure.

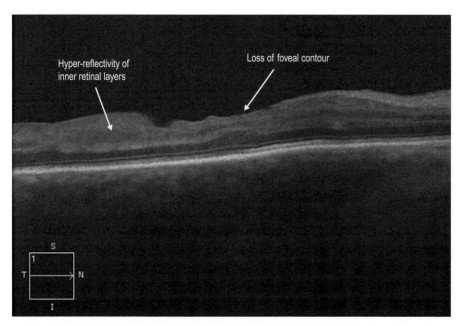

Figure 18.5.2 OCT (corresponding to Figure 18.5.1) shows significant, subclinical, disease activity that is evident within the macula. Abnormal hyper-reflectivity within the inner retinal layers is a sign of active disease. There is also loss of the normal foveal contour.

PART 7: Trauma

19.1 | Commotio Retinae

Introduction: Commotio retinae or Berlin's edema occurs in the setting of non-penetrating, blunt globe trauma. It may affect any area of the retina and is generally self-limited, but when the macula is involved visual acuity may be permanently decreased.

Clinical Features: There is retinal whitening due to damage of the outer retinal layers. The whitening is generally patchy with ill-defined borders and does not follow a vascular distribution (Fig. 19.1.1).

OCT Features: When involving the macula, acutely, there is obscuration of the retinal layers in the involved region with **disruption of the IS–OS/ellipsoid zone and retinal pigment epithelium inter-digitation**, sometimes leaving a **cleft of empty hyporeflective space** under the neurosensory retina (Fig. 19.1.2). There can be a hyper-reflective signal throughout the retinal layers, but this tends to be most pronounced in the **outer layers**. Later, the retina can return to normal in mild cases, or there may be permanent loss of outer retina including photoreceptors and the retinal pigment epithelium in severe cases (Fig. 19.1.3).

Ancillary Testing: No ancillary testing is generally required.

Treatment: Most cases are self-limiting, but in severe cases, where visual damage can occur, no treatment has proven efficacy.

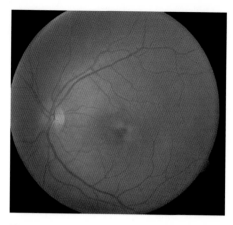

Figure 19.1.1 Color fundus photograph of commotio retinae involving the central macula. Retinal whitening is visible in the affected region.

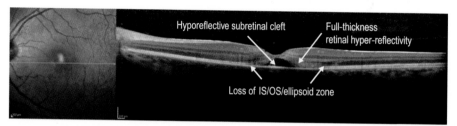

Figure 19.1.2 OCT in the acute setting of commotio retinae shows loss of the IS–OS/ellipsoid zone (between arrow heads) with overlying outer retinal hyper-reflectivity. There is a subretinal cleft of empty, hyporeflective space with surrounding full-thickness retinal hyper-reflectivity.

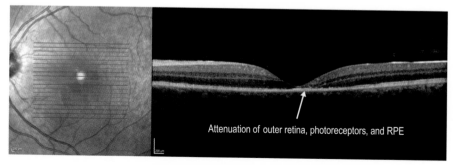

Figure 19.1.3 OCT in the chronic setting of severe commotio retinae shows attenuation of the outer retina, photoreceptors, and RPE.

Introduction: Choroidal ruptures occur following blunt trauma severe enough to cause significant globe compression with subsequent rupture of Bruch's membrane, RPE, and the inner choroid.

Clinical Features: Choroidal ruptures typically occur concentrically to the optic nerve, most commonly temporally and involving the macula (Fig. 19.2.1 and Fig. 19.2.2). There is usually associated hemorrhage in the acute setting, which may be intraretinal or subretinal in location. Over time, the hemorrhage will clear, leaving an arc-shaped area of subretinal de-pigmentation with clumps of hyperpigmentation. Secondary CNV can occur months or years after trauma resulting in further visual loss.

OCT Features: In the acute setting, associated hemorrhage often obscures the presence of a choroidal rupture from view with OCT. As the hemorrhage clears, it becomes more visible and more easily imaged. In the acute or subacute setting, a choroidal rupture appears as an **elevated, nodule-like abnormality spanning Bruch's membrane, the RPE, and inner choroid** (Figs 19.2.3). With time, the nodular abnormality flattens, leaving a noticeably deformed area that exhibits **negative shadowing** from focal loss of the RPE (Fig. 19.2.4 and 19.2.5).

Ancillary Testing: Fluorescein angiography and/or indocyanine green angiography can be helpful in identifying the presence of a choroidal rupture site (Fig. 19.2.2) if the diagnosis is in question. FA can also be helpful to evaluate for the presence of an associated CNV membrane, which can develop later in up to 10% of eyes.

Treatment: In the absence of CNV, observation alone is generally advocated. If CNV is present, intravitreal anti-vascular endothelial growth factor therapy is indicated.

FIGURE LEGENDS

Figure 19.2.1 Color photograph of two separate choroidal rupture sites (arrowheads) and shallow overlying subretinal hemorrhage two weeks following blunt trauma. *(Courtesy of Jeffrey S. Heier, MD.)*

Figure 19.2.2 Fluorescein angiography shows hyperfluorescence due to window defects in the location of the two choroidal rupture sites. *(Courtesy of Jeffrey S. Heier, MD.)*

Figure 19.2.3 OCT through two separate choroidal rupture sites two weeks following injury. Overlying subretinal hemorrhage is also present. *(Courtesy of Jeffrey S. Heier, MD.)*

Figure 19.2.4 OCT through the same choroidal rupture sites, one month following injury, shows a decrease in size of the nodule-like elevations spanning Bruch's membrane, the retinal pigment epithelium, and inner choroid. *(Courtesy of Jeffrey S. Heier, MD.)*

Figure 19.2.5 OCT through the same choroidal rupture sites, three months following injury, shows a continued flattening of the choroidal rupture sites. There is negative shadowing due to focal loss of retinal pigment epithelium that is highlighted (between arrowheads). *(Courtesy of Jeffrey S. Heier, MD.)*

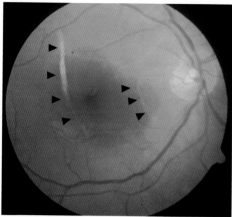
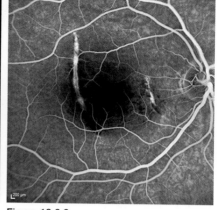

Figure 19.2.1

Figure 19.2.2

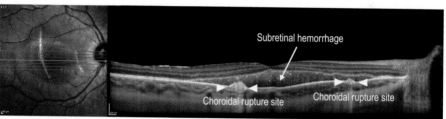

Subretinal hemorrhage

Choroidal rupture site   Choroidal rupture site

Figure 19.2.3

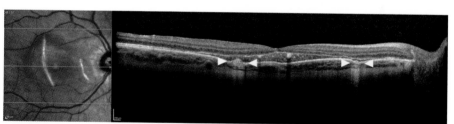

Figure 19.2.4

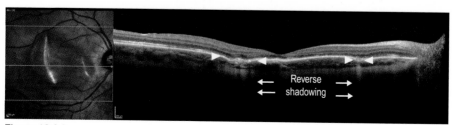

Reverse shadowing

Figure 19.2.5

19.3 | Valsalva Retinopathy

Introduction: Valsalva retinopathy results from a sudden increase in intraocular venous pressure due to forced exhalation against a closed glottis. This leads to rupture of superficial capillaries in predisposed individuals.

Clinical Features: Preretinal hemorrhage accumulates in the sub-internal limiting membrane space, typically overlying the macula (Fig. 19.3.1). With rest, the red blood cells layer such that there is a serous component superiorly.

OCT Features: The **superior** serous component forms a **hyporeflective cavity** (Fig. 19.3.2), whereas the **inferior** hemorrhagic component forms a **hyper-reflective cavity** that blocks the underlying structures (Fig. 19.3.3). OCT can confirm the specific location of the hemorrhage, such as in the sub-internal limiting membrane space (Fig. 19.3.4). OCT is also helpful to monitor the progression and resolution of hemorrhage over time (Fig. 19.3.5).

Ancillary Testing: Fluorescein angiography and indocyanine green angiography can be used to rule out mimicking lesions like macroaneurysms, choroidal neovascularization, or idiopathic polypoidal choroidal vasculopathy.

Treatment: Observation is most typically recommended. Nd:YAG laser membranotomy and surgical evacuation are options in select cases.

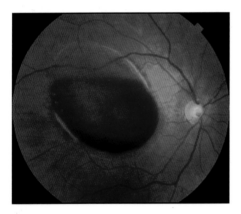

Figure 19.3.1 Color photograph of valsalva retinopathy with a layered pre-macular hemorrhage. *(Modified from Goldman, D.R. & Baumal, C.R. Natural history of valsalva retinopathy in an adolescent. Journal of Pediatric Ophthalmology and Strabismus, in press.)*

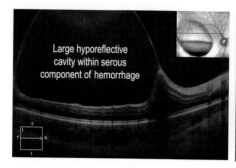

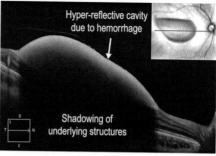

Figure 19.3.2 Horizontal line scan OCT through the superior serous component (corresponding to Figure 1) shows a large hyporeflective cavity. *(Modified from Goldman, D.R. & Baumal, C.R. Natural history of valsalva retinopathy in an adolescent. Journal of Pediatric Ophthalmology and Strabismus, in press.)*

Figure 19.3.3 Horizontal line scan OCT through the inferior hemorrhagic component (corresponding to Figure 19.3.1) shows a large hyper-reflective cavity. *(Modified from Goldman, D.R. & Baumal, C.R. Natural history of valsalva retinopathy in an adolescent. Journal of Pediatric Ophthalmology and Strabismus, in press.)*

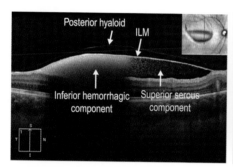

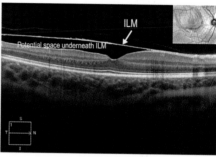

Figure 19.3.4 Vertical line scan OCT shows both the superior serous and inferior hemorrhagic components. Individual red blood cells can be seen disbursed within the serous component. The pre-macular hemorrhage is located underneath the internal limiting membrane. The posterior hyaloid face can also be seen. ILM, internal limiting membrane. *(Modified from Goldman, D.R. & Baumal, C.R. Natural history of valsalva retinopathy in an adolescent. Journal of Pediatric Ophthalmology and Strabismus, in press.)*

Figure 19.3.5 Upon resolution of the hemorrhage, a potential space underneath the internal limiting membrane (ILM) is still present. *(Modified from Goldman, D.R. & Baumal, C.R. Natural history of valsalva retinopathy in an adolescent. Journal of Pediatric Ophthalmology and Strabismus, in press.)*

20.1 Laser Injury (Photothermal and Photomechanical)

Introduction: Accidental laser injuries to the retina are uncommon, but can occur with photo-thermal injury (typically high-powered handheld laser pointers) and/or photomechanical injury (typically research and military devices).

Clinical Features: The affected region of the retina is typically the central macula. In the acute setting, laser injuries produce a yellow subretinal lesion that can be of varied appearance (Fig. 20.1.1). Within a short time, the affected area becomes pigmented and over time this appearance can resolve leaving more subtle retinal pigment epithelium disturbances.

OCT Features: A significant photothermal laser injury causes retinal trauma identical to photo-coagulation. On OCT, this is seen as **localized outer retinal, IS–OS/ellipsoid zone, and RPE disruption** in the acute setting (Figs 20.1.2 and 20.1.3). The inner retina may also be affected (Fig. 20.1.4). With mild exposure, the findings may be very subtle (Fig. 20.1.5). The abnormalities tend to **fade quickly**, in most cases, over weeks to months (Figs 20.1.6 and 20.1.7).

Ancillary Testing: Fluorescein angiography can be helpful to evaluate for the presence of any associated choroidal neovascularization.

Treatment: As these injuries are very rare, no therapy has been proven to have definite efficacy though oral corticosteroids have been used in the acute setting.

FIGURE LEGENDS

Figure 20.1.1 Color photograph shows yellow subretinal deposits in a splotchy pattern within the central macula. This patient was exposed to a high-powered handheld class 3B laser pointer.

Figure 20.1.2 OCT (corresponding to Figure 20.1.1) shows focal disruption of the outer retina, ELM, IS–OS/ellipsoid zone, and RPE underlying the fovea. There is also a thin hyporeflective empty space above the focal disruption.

Figure 20.1.3 OCT of a different accidental high-powered laser pointer injury also shows focal disruption of the outer retina, ELM, IS–OS/ellipsoid zone, and RPE with a collection of hyper-reflective material under the retina.

Figure 20.1.4 OCT of an accidental military defense laser injury shows an abnormal hyper-reflective signal involving the full thickness of the retina in the fovea.

There is also a tiny pocket of subretinal fluid adjacent to the central abnormality.

Figure 20.1.5 OCT of the fellow eye of the patient in Figure 20.1.2 shows a subtle abnormality due to limited exposure of this eye to the laser beam. There is a vertical, linear, hyper-reflective abnormality underneath the center of the fovea that spans from the RPE to the external limiting membrane.

Figure 20.1.6 One month following the injury (see Figure 20.1.3), OCT shows near resolution of the focal outer retinal disruption and subretinal material. The IS–OS/ellipsoid zone and RPE are still somewhat attenuated underneath the fovea.

Figure 20.1.7 One month following the injury (see Figure 20.1.4), OCT shows shrinking of the focal outer retinal disruption underneath the fovea and the inner retinal hyper-reflective signal has resolved.

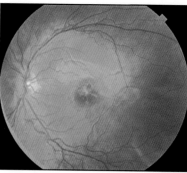

Figure 20.1.1

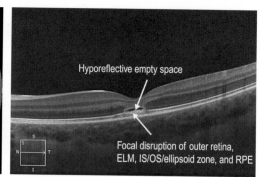

Hyporeflective empty space

Focal disruption of outer retina,
ELM, IS/OS/ellipsoid zone, and RPE

Figure 20.1.2

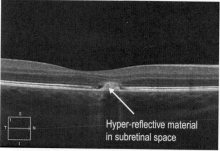

Hyper-reflective material
in subretinal space

Figure 20.1.3

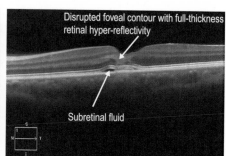

Disrupted foveal contour with full-thickness
retinal hyper-reflectivity

Subretinal fluid

Figure 20.1.4

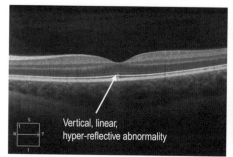

Vertical, linear,
hyper-reflective abnormality

Figure 20.1.5

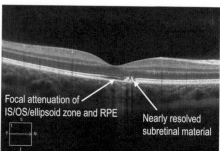

Focal attenuation of
IS/OS/ellipsoid zone and RPE

Nearly resolved
subretinal material

Figure 20.1.6

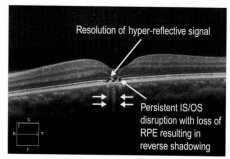

Resolution of hyper-reflective signal

Persistent IS/OS
disruption with loss of
RPE resulting in
reverse shadowing

Figure 20.1.7

20.2 | Retinal Light Toxicity (Photochemical)

Introduction: Accidental light-induced injuries to the retina from a photochemical mechanism can occur from prolonged exposure to the sun, from a welding arc, and from intra-operative microscope illumination.

Clinical Features: Retinal phototoxicity from the sun or a welding arc appears as small, round, well-circumscribed, yellow acquired vitelliform-like lesions in the fovea (Fig. 20.2.1). Microscope phototoxicity appears as a more broad area that is fairly well-circumscribed either in the inferior or superior macula (dependent on tilt of microscope).

OCT Features: Solar and welding arc injuries appear similar on OCT as a **focal loss of the outer retina** and **IS–OS/ellipsoid layer**, leaving a small **hyporeflective rectangular cavity** or outer retinal hole (Fig. 20.2.2). These can be singular or multifocal. The ELM and RPE are typically spared. Microscope light-induced retinal phototoxicity leads to prominent chorioretinal scarring in the region of the injury.

Ancillary Testing: Fluorescein angiography can show a pinpoint window defect centrally in solar retinopathy, but no other imaging modality is as useful as OCT.

Treatment: No treatment is available, but avoidance of additional pathologic light exposure is recommended.

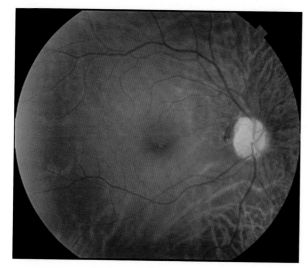

Figure 20.2.1 Color fundus photograph of solar retinal phototoxicity shows a small, central, ovoid light-colored abnormality with a hyper-pigmented rim located in the fovea.

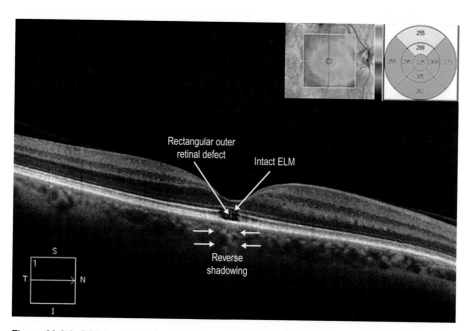

Figure 20.2.2 OCT (corresponding to Figure 20.2.1) shows focal loss of the outer retina including photoreceptors and the IS–OS/ellipsoid layer. In this advanced case, the RPE is also affected, leading to 'reverse shadowing' below (between arrowheads). The overall defect is characteristically rectangle-shaped and the overlying ELM is intact.

PART 8: Tumors

21.1 Choroidal Nevus

Introduction: Choroidal nevi are common, acquired lesions that are typically discovered during routine funduscopic examination in the absence of symptoms.

Clinical Features: They are typically darkly pigmented, small, flat, and with well-defined borders (Fig. 21.1.1). Overlying drusen, present in Bruch's membrane, are a common finding. Some nevi may have slight elevation (Fig. 21.1.2). They can occur throughout the fundus but are usually seen in the posterior pole. Accumulation of subretinal fluid, minimal growth over time, and alterations in pigmentation can occur in the absence of malignant transformation.

OCT Features: There is loss of the features of the choroicapillaris in the area of the nevus, which appears as a homogeneous well-defined area of hyper-reflectivity below the RPE (Figs 21.1.3 and 21.1.4). The overlying retinal layers are undisturbed. Enhanced depth imaging techniques can help to visualize the more posterior extent of a choroidal nevus (Fig. 21.1.5).

Ancillary Testing: B-scan ultrasonography can be used to determine if the lesion is elevated to help in distinguishing this lesion from a choroidal melanoma.

Treatment: No treatment is typically necessary. Serial observation is recommended.

FIGURE LEGENDS

Figure 21.1.1 Wide-angle image of a flat nevus shows a darkly pigmented, well-circumscribed flat choroidal lesion in the superior macula.

Figure 21.1.2 Color fundus photograph of a minimally elevated nevus shows a darkly pigmented, well-circumscribed choroidal lesion in the inferior mid-periphery. There is overlying drusen present.

Figure 21.1.3 OCT (corresponding to Figure 21.1.1) shows a homogeneous, well-defined area of hyper-reflectivity below the RPE that obscures the features of the choriocapillaris in this region, corresponding to the choroidal nevus (arrows).

Figure 21.1.4 OCT (corresponding to Figure 21.1.2) shows a homogeneous well-defined area of hyper-reflectivity below the RPE that obscures the features of the underlying choriocapillaris centrally, but blends with the choriocapillaris on the edges. The overlying retina has a mild dome-shaped elevation due to the height of the lesion.

Figure 21.1.5 OCT with enhanced depth imaging shows the edges of a flat nevus more clearly. The underlying structures are obscured by shadowing.

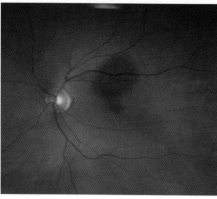
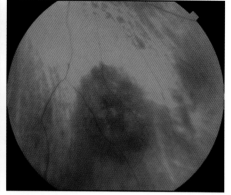

Figure 21.1.1

Figure 21.1.2

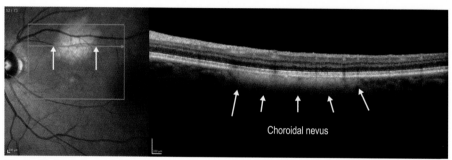

Figure 21.1.3

Choroidal nevus

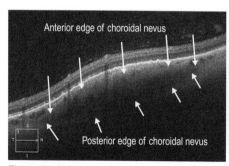

Anterior edge of choroidal nevus

Posterior edge of choroidal nevus

Figure 21.1.4

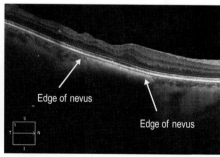

Edge of nevus

Edge of nevus

Figure 21.1.5

21.2 | Choroidal Melanoma

Introduction: Choroidal melanoma is the most common primary intraocular malignancy in adults, but is still quite rare with an incidence of about six per one million people. It most commonly presents in the sixth decade, but can affect individuals of any age. In most studied populations, there is a slight predisposition towards males.

Clinical Features: The most common appearance is a pigmented, elevated choroidal lesion that will enlarge without treatment (Fig. 21.2.1 and Fig. 21.2.2). Without documented growth, features such as overlying lipofuscin (orange pigment), associated subretinal fluid, larger size, and proximity to the optic nerve help to differentiate from benign lesions such as choroidal nevus. On a clinical basis, the diagnosis can be made with greater than 99% accuracy. Biopsy is rarely necessary, but can confirm the diagnosis. Radiation retinopathy can often develop after treatment with external radiation (Fig 21.2.3).

OCT Features: A large homogeneous **hyporeflective, elevated area of choroidal infiltration** is typically seen in association with **overlying subretinal fluid** (Figs. 21.2.4 and 21.2.5). Enhanced depth imaging OCT can assist the documentation of relatively small melanomas. Older lesions can exhibit cystoid retinal degeneration over the surface of the tumor. More acute lesions can show shaggy photoreceptors overlying subretinal fluid. Associated retinopathy can lead to severe **cystoid macular edema** and retinal atrophy (Fig. 21.2.6).

Ancillary Testing: B-scan ultrasonography can be useful in distinguishing choroidal melanoma from benign lesions, such as choroidal nevus. Fluorescein angiography can also be helpful by demonstrating a characteristic internal circulation within the melanoma (Fig. 21.2.2).

Treatment: Radiation therapy (plaque brachytherapy, proton beam, gamma knife) is the most common treatment approach, with enucleation generally reserved for very large and advanced tumors with poor visual prognosis. Post-radiation retinopathy is not uncommon, which can be difficult to treat, but is sometimes responsive to focal laser photocoagulation and/or intravitreal anti-vascular endothelial growth factor therapy.

FIGURE LEGENDS

Figure 21.2.1 Color fundus photograph of a large, elevated pigmented choroidal melanoma. The lesion is so elevated that the neighboring macula and optic nerve are out of focus.

Figure 21.2.2 Late phase fluorescein angiogram (corresponding to Figure 21.2.1) shows an internal circulation of the choroidal melanoma.

Figure 21.2.3 Color fundus photograph of radiation retinopathy following I-125 plaque brachytherapy for choroidal melanoma. Optic disc edema, intraretinal hemorrhages, cystoid macular edema, and hard exudates are all present.

Figure 21.2.4 OCT (corresponding to Figure 21.2.1) shows a large hyporeflective cavity in the choroidal space corresponding to the melanoma with adjacent subretinal fluid. There

is mirror artifact overlying the hyporeflective cavity on the left side of the image. There is shadowing underneath the melanoma blocking the choroid and sclera.

Figure 21.2.5 OCT of another choroidal melanoma with a large hyporeflective cavity in the choroidal space that is elevating the overlying retina. There is a cap of subretinal fluid overlying the lesion and additional hyper-reflective material in the subretinal space, which may represent shed photorecepters. The inner retina is abnormally hyper-reflective.

Figure 21.2.6 OCT (corresponding to Figure 21.2.2) shows severe cystoid macular edema (CME) with adjacent retinal atrophy. There is also generalized loss of photoreceptors.

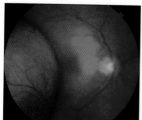

Figure 21.2.1

Figure 21.2.2

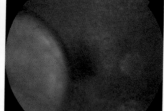

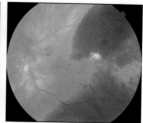

Figure 21.2.3

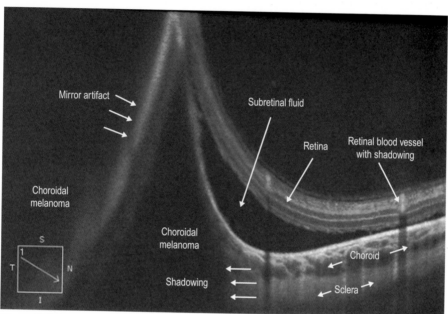

Figure 21.2.4

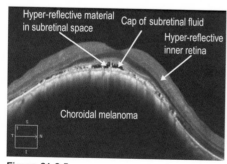

Figure 21.2.5

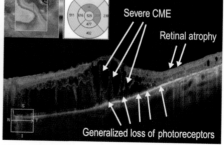

Figure 21.2.6

21.3 | Choroidal Hemangioma

Introduction: Choroidal hemangiomas are benign vascular tumors that present in two distinct forms:
- Solitary (circumscribed)
- Diffuse

The solitary lesions are most commonly an isolated finding, while the diffuse form is rare and typically associated with Sturge–Weber syndrome.

Clinical Features: They may be identified as an incidental finding, but can affect visual acuity if there is associated subretinal fluid or cystic fluid involving the macula. Typical features include a reddish/orange coloration and location in the posterior pole (Fig. 21.3.1). RPE metaplasia on the surface is not rare. Occasionally, clinical findings are subtle and they are only identified on OCT.

OCT Features: There is obscuration of the normal choriocapillaris by a hyporeflective signal and overlying round-shaped retinal elevation (Figs 21.3.2 and 21.3.3). Overlying subretinal and/or intraretinal fluid may also be present (Fig. 21.3.3), which can involve the macula (Fig. 21.3.4). Occasionally, fluid can occur subfoveally, even if the tumor is not located within the macula. Enhanced depth imaging techniques can be helpful for better visualization in larger tumors.

Ancillary Testing: Indocyanine green angiography is useful in confirming the diagnosis, particularly in the early phase images 20–30 seconds following injection where prominent hyperfluorescence of the lesion is noted (Fig. 21.3.5). B-scan ultrasonography can also be helpful.

Treatment: If visual acuity is affected by the presence of subretinal fluid in the macula, photodynamic therapy is the most commonly used therapy, though various other treatments have been used.

FIGURE LEGENDS

Figure 21.3.1 Color photograph of a clinically evident choroidal hemagioma (arrowheads). There are associated retinal striae and the foveal reflex is blunted due to the presence of subretinal fluid.

Figure 21.3.5 Indocyanine green angiography at 20 seconds (corresponding to Figure 21.3.1) shows intense early hyperfluorescence of the choroidal hemangioma, which is a characteristic feature distinguishing this lesion from other choroidal tumors.

Figure 21.3.2 OCT of a subtle choroidal hemangioma that was not clearly visible clinically. The choriocapillaris is slightly obscured (abnormal hyporeflectivity between arrowheads) and there is elevation of the overlying retina.

Figure 21.3.3 OCT of a more obvious choroidal hemangioma (corresponding to Figure 21.3.1). The choriocapillaris is completely obscured by the tumor and there is bullous overlying retinal elevation. Subretinal and intraretinal fluid are also present.

Figure 21.3.4 OCT of the macula (corresponding to Figure 21.3.3) shows the presence of subretinal fluid and a mild epiretinal membrane.

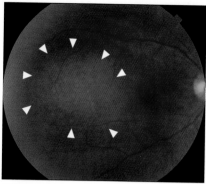

Figure 21.3.1

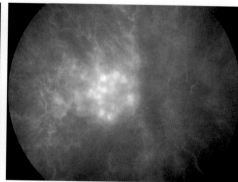

Figure 21.3.5

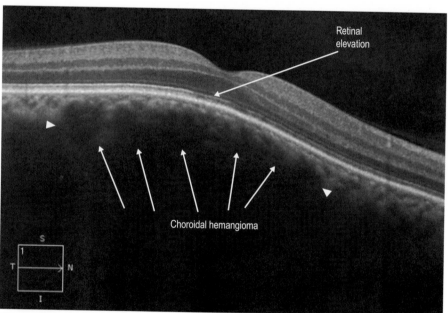

Retinal elevation

Choroidal hemangioma

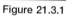

Figure 21.3.2

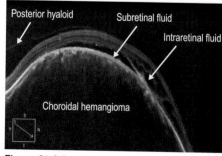

Posterior hyaloid

Subretinal fluid

Intraretinal fluid

Choroidal hemangioma

Figure 21.3.3

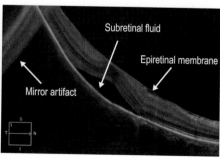

Subretinal fluid

Epiretinal membrane

Mirror artifact

Figure 21.3.4

22.1 | Retinal Capillary Hemangioma

Introduction: Retinal capillary hemangiomas (RCH), or hemangioblastomas, are usually seen in association with Von Hippel–Lindau disease, but can also occur sporadically.

Clinical Features: These lesions can affect both the retina and optic nerve. They start out small and can gradually enlarge with the possibility of intraretinal and subretinal exudation that can involve the macula and affect visual acuity. They have characteristic tortuous and dilated feeding and draining arteries and veins (Fig. 22.1.1 and Fig. 22.1.2), respectively. Multiple and bilateral lesions are common in the setting of Von Hippel–Lindau disease.

OCT Features: Smaller lesions are seen as a **well-circumscribed** bulbous deformity **obscuring the layers of the retina** (Fig. 22.1.3), whereas larger lesions have a **hyper-reflective inner surface** with deeper structures obscured by shadowing (Fig. 22.1.4). In larger lesions with surrounding exudation, there can be cystic cavities within the retina surrounding the retinal angioma (Fig. 22.1.5). There can be associated intraretinal fluid or even a serous retinal detachment within the macula (Fig. 22.1.6).

Ancillary Testing: Serial color, red free photos and ultrasonography can be helpful in tracking changes in lesion size over time. Fluorescein angiography can also be useful in assisting with the diagnosis (Fig. 22.1.2), if it is in question.

Treatment: In general, lesions that are not leaking can be observed. Once peripheral lesions begin to leak, treatment is usually contemplated. Due to the possibility of collateral damage to the optic disc, lesions on the nerve are typically watched until moderate visual loss occurs. Various albative techniques can be used for therapy, depending on size and location of the lesions, including photodynamic therapy, laser photocoagulation, and cryotherapy.

FIGURE LEGENDS

Figure 22.1.1 Color fundus photograph of a retinal capillary hemangioma shows a pink-colored lesion just superior to the macula with dilated and tortuous feeding vessels. There is surrounding subretinal fluid and exudation present.

Figure 22.1.2 Late phase FA of a retinal capillary hemangioma shows bright hyperfluorescence of the lesion and highlights the feeding vasculature.

Figure 22.1.3 OCT of a smaller peripheral RCH shows a well-circumscribed area of hyper-reflectivity corresponding to the lesion that focally replaces the retina. The underlying choroid appears thin, though there is significant shadowing artifact.

Figure 22.1.4 OCT of a large RCH shows hyper-reflectivity of the inner surface with a dense shadowing artifact of the central and outer portions. There is mild CME on the edges.

Figure 22.1.5 OCT of a large retinal capillary hemangioma (corresponding to Figure 22.1.1) shows significant hyper-reflectivity of the inner surface (between arrowheads). There is also significant surrounding intraretinal fluid or CME.

Figure 22.1.6 OCT of the macula in a patient with a peripheral retinal capillary hemangioma shows significant CME and a sizeable serous retinal detachment. Hard exudates are also present within the henle fiber layer (or axonal outer plexiform layer).

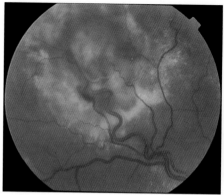

Figure 22.1.1

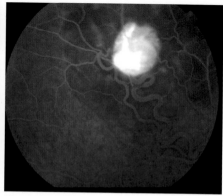

Figure 22.1.2

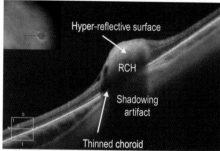

Figure 22.1.3

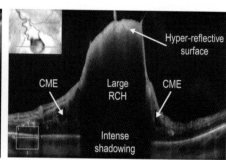

Figure 22.1.4

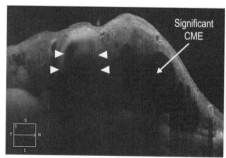

Figure 22.1.5

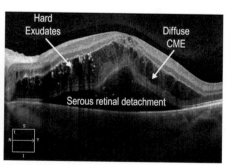

Figure 22.1.6

22.2 | Retinoblastoma

Introduction: Retinoblastoma is the most common pediatric intraocular malignancy, representing about 5% of all pediatric malignancies.

Clinical Features: The most common presenting feature is leukocoria, but others include strabismus, decreased vision, and a painful eye. Characteristic clinical features include a white or yellow-white elevated, fungating, singular or multifocal retinal tumor (Fig. 22.2.1). Associated vitreous and subretinal seeding may also be present.

OCT Features: OCT shows involvement of the neurosensory retina, particularly the **photoreceptors** and **outer retina**. Early in tumor growth or along the leading edge of the tumor, these features can be more clearly seen (Fig. 22.2.2). In larger or more advanced tumors, the entire **neurosensory retina can be obscured** but the underlying **retinal pigment epithelial layer is preserved** (Figs 22.2.3 and 22.2.4).

Ancillary Testing: Fluorescein angiography may be helpful to differentiate from other simulating lesions such as Coats disease, toxocariasis, or retinal astrocytoma. Radiography and/or ultrasonography characteristically show internal calcification. Trans-scleral or trans-pars plana biopsy are contraindicated because of the risk of initiating metastasis.

Treatment: Treatment options include intravenous chemotherapy, intra-arterial chemotherapy, cryotherapy, laser photocoagulation, external radiation, and enucleation. The specific treatment is individualized to the unique patient condition.

FIGURE LEGENDS

Figure 22.2.1 Color photograph of retinoblastoma in an infant shows two separate lesions involving the posterior pole of differing sizes. Both are round, elevated, and creamy-white in color. *(Courtesy of Carol Shields, MD.)*

Figure 22.2.2 OCT (corresponding to line mark section of the scan in Figure 22.2.1) shows the edge of the tumor located above the RPE and involving the outer retina. The tumor appears to be arising from the photoreceptor layer. The central fovea is uninvolved. *(Courtesy of Carol Shields, MD.)*

Figure 22.2.3 OCT (corresponding to Figure 22.2.1, horizontal scan through macular lesion) shows a fairly homogeneous hyper-reflective mass that has obliterated the retinal layers completely. The transition to partial involvement of the retina and normal retina can also be seen. *(Courtesy of Carol Shields, MD.)*

Figure 22.2.4 OCT (corresponding to Figure 22.2.1, vertical scan through macular lesion) illustrates that the underlying RPE layer is intact and not involved (arrowheads). *(Courtesy of Carol Shields, MD.)*

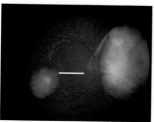

Figure 22.2.1

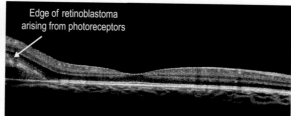

Figure 22.2.2

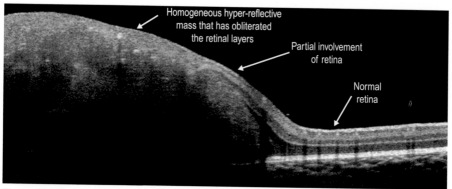

Figure 22.2.3

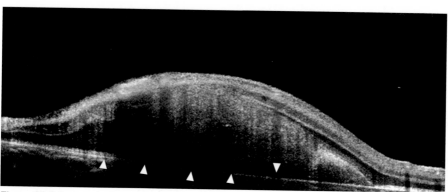

Figure 22.2.4

23.1 | Metastatic Choroidal Tumor

Introduction: Choroidal metastatic lesions are the most common intraocular tumor in adults. The most common primary sites are breast and lung.

Clinical Features: These lesions are typically creamy, yellow, and elevated. They tend to be bilateral and can also be multifocal (Fig. 23.1.1). Associated serous retinal detachments can cause decreased visual acuity when involving the macula. A history of primary malignancy is helpful in confirming the diagnosis.

OCT Features: There is a localized elevation of the choroid in the location of the tumor, which can have overlying subretinal fluid (Fig. 23.1.2). Cystoid intraretinal fluid overlying the tumor can also be present (Figs 23.1.3 and 23.1.4).

Ancillary Testing: Ultrasonography is particularly helpful in providing supportive evidence to the diagnosis with metastatic choroidal lesions typically displaying moderate to high internal reflectivity. Fluorescein angiography is not that helpful in differentiation from primary choroidal tumors.

Treatment: The need for local treatment depends on the type and extent of metastatic lesions as many respond adequately to systemic chemotherapy. Any of the various external radiation modalities can be used as adjunctive therapy, when necessary.

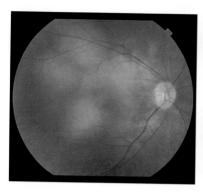

Figure 23.1.1 Color fundus photo shows numerous creamy, yellowish, circular, minimally elevated choroidal tumors within the posterior pole in a patient with pulmonary metastases.

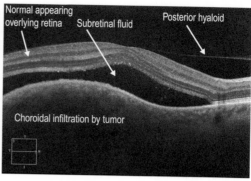

Figure 23.1.2 OCT (corresponding to Figure 23.1.1) shows a hill-like elevation of the choroid due to infiltration by the tumor with mild obscuration of the choriocapillaris. There is overlying subretinal fluid.

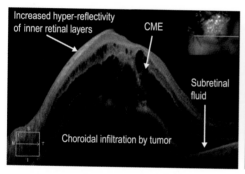

Figure 23.1.3 OCT of a large metastatic choroidal tumor involving the optic nerve and macula shows a hyporeflective elevation of the choroid that is infiltrated by tumor. Overlying this is subretinal fluid and extensive CME. The inner retinal layers are somewhat more hyper-reflective than normal.

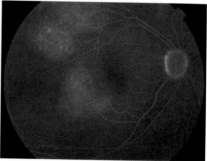

Figure 23.1.4 Fluorescein angiography (corresponding to Figure 23.1.1) shows multiple areas of pinpoint hyperfluorescence overlying each area of choroidal infiltration.

23.2 | Vitreoretinal Lymphoma

Introduction: Primary vitreoretinal lymphoma (VRL) is an uncommon form of primary central nervous system lymphoma. Typically it is a malignant B-cell non-Hodgkin lymphoma. Ninety per cent of affected patients eventually develop concurrent central nervous system involvement. The prognosis for survival historically has been poor but more recently seems to be improving.

Clinical Features: There are no clinical pathognomonic features of VRL and confirmation of the diagnosis can be difficult as it typically presents as an unspecified posterior uveitis. In certain cases, lymphoma cells can invade the subretinal space, leading to characteristic multifocal, dome-shaped yellowish subretinal deposits. These can be located within the macula, but are most striking when located in the retinal periphery (Fig. 23.2.1).

OCT Features: The lymphoma cells infiltrate along Bruch's membrane and accumulate as deposits underneath the RPE. These deposits appear on OCT as medium to intense hyper-reflective dome-shaped sub-RPE elevations of varying size. They can be seen both in the macula (Fig. 23.2.2) and retinal periphery (Fig. 23.2.3).

Ancillary Testing: Fluorescein angiography may reveal a leopard spot pattern. A vitrectomy to obtain a diagnostic sample is often necessary to confirm the diagnosis. Pathologic studies employed to confirm the diagnosis include: cytology, immunohistochemistry, flow cytometry, polymerase chain reaction analysis of the immunoglobulin heavy chain gene rearrangement (B-cell lymphoma) and T-cell receptor gene clonality (T-cell lymphoma), IL-10/IL-6 ratio and kappa chain evaluation.

Treatment: Consultation with an oncologist should be undertaken if VRL is suspected. A combination of radiation and systemic chemotherapy are the mainstay of treatment. Intravitreal chemotherapy (methotrexate, rituximab) can be used as adjunctive therapy, particularly when systemic toxicity is an issue.

FIGURE LEGENDS

Figure 23.2.1   Color photograph of vitreoretinal lymphoma shows numerous creamy nodular sub-RPE elevations (arrows). Smaller lesions are located in the macula, whereas larger lesions are located in the nasal periphery.

Figure 23.2.2   OCT (corresponding to Figure 23.2.1, macula) shows a small sub-RPE nodular elevation that exhibits hyper-reflectivity of medium intensity (arrow). This nodule is believed to be composed of lymphoma cells.

Figure 23.2.3   OCT (corresponding to Figure 23.2.1, nasal periphery) shows numerous, large sub-RPE nodular elevations, which are underneath the neurosensory retina. These lesions are intensely hyper-reflective.

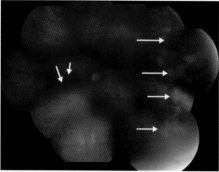

Figure 23.2.1

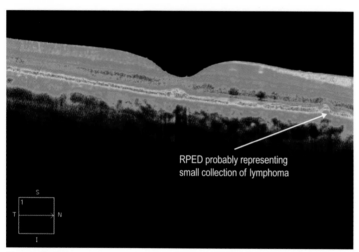

RPED probably representing
small collection of lymphoma

Figure 23.2.2

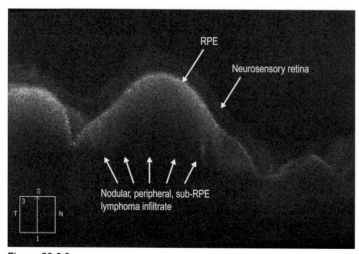

RPE

Neurosensory retina

Nodular, peripheral, sub-RPE
lymphoma infiltrate

Figure 23.2.3

PART 9: Peripheral Retinal Abnormalities

24.1 Retinal Detachment

Introduction: Retinal detachment (RD) is a separation of the neurosensory retina from the underlying retinal pigment epithelium. There are three different forms of RDs:
- Rhegmatogenous
- Exudative
- Tractional.

Some eyes may present with a combination of these three. Tractional and exudative detachments are dealt in greater detail in the chapters associated with their underlying pathologies. Rhegmatogenous RD are more common in men, particularly those between 40 and 70 years of age. Risk factors for rhegmatogenous RD include prior cataract surgery, myopia, trauma, peripheral lattice degeneration, a family history of rhegmatogenous RDs, retinal tears and other intraocular surgery. Tractional RDs occur most commonly in the setting of fibrous membranes in the vitreous, secondary to diseases like proliferative diabetic retinopathy, retinopathy of prematurity, sickle cell retinopathy, trauma or proliferative vitreoretinopathy. Exudative RDs occur secondary to neoplastic or inflammatory processes, central serous chorioretinopathy, or uveal effusion syndrome

Clinical features: Patients with rhegmatogenous RD present with painless unilateral decrease in vision or visual field with flashes and floaters. Most eyes have a posterior vitreous detachment. Examination reveals elevation of the retina, with a corrugated appearance and generally clear subretinal fluid that does not shift with position. The pathognomonic sign of a rhegmatogenous RD is the presence of one or more retinal tears or full thickness holes (Fig. 24.1.1).

Exudative RDs are serous, with a smooth surface and with shifting subretinal fluid. Other signs may be seen depending on the etiology.

Tractional RDs show preretinal proliferation with traction on the retinal surface and elevated, taut retina.

OCT Features: OCT of RD shows **elevation of the neurosensory retina** from the underlying RPE (Figs 24.1.2 and 24.1.3). No splitting of retinal layers is seen except in the setting of combined retinoschisis-rhegmatogenous RD. Occasionally, RDs especially chronic RDs may be associated with **cystic changes** within the retina. The subretinal fluid in rhegmatogenous RDs is usually **clear** and **hyporeflective**.

Tractional RDs show **hyper-reflective bands** that attach to the inner retina and cause retinal elevation.

Serous RDs may occasionally be associated with **turbid subretinal fluid** that is hyper-reflective.

Ancillary Testing: The diagnosis of rhegmatogenous RDs is made on clinical examination. Tractional and serous RDs may need additional testing based on the underlying pathophysiology. B-scan ultrasonography is critical in the setting of cloudy media.

Management: Rhegmatogenous RD usually require surgical intervention, with pneumatic retinopexy, vitrectomy surgery or scleral buckling surgery, or a combination of both. Laser demarcation is an option in peripheral rhegmatogenous RD.

The management of tractional and serous RDs depends on their underlying etiology and the location of the detachment in relation to the macula.

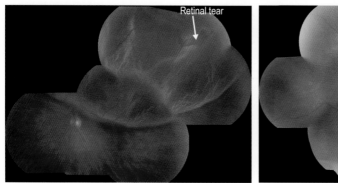
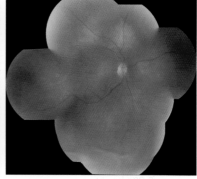

Figure 24.1.1 Color photograph shows a rhegmatogenous retinal detachment with a retinal tear. Note the corrugated, transparent retinal surface. The second photograph shows a serous retinal detachment.

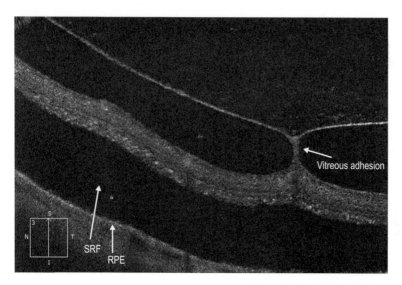

Figure 24.1.2 OCT scan through a retinal detachment shows separation of the neurosensory retina from the hyper-reflective underlying RPE. There is SRF seen. Note the site of vitreous attachment on the retina.

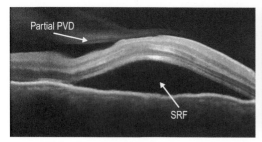
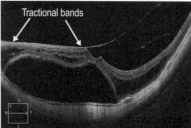

Figure 24.1.3 OCT scan through a serous retinal detachment on the left and a tractional detachment on the right. Note the smooth surface of the serous detachment and the preretinal fibrous tractional bands and hyaloidal thickening in the tractional retinal detachment.

25.1 Retinoschisis

Introduction: Retinoschisis is defined as splitting of the retinal layers. In the peripheral retina, it occurs in a senile (more common) and a juvenile X-linked form. Traction on the macula can induce macular retinoschisis as well. This is most commonly seen in highly myopic individuals but rarely can occur secondary to an ERM or in an otherwise normal eye. Senile retinoschisis is estimated to occur in 4% of eyes of normal individuals. There is no gender preponderance. Most are stable and chronic, but some (around 1%) may progress to retinal detachment after developing inner and outer retinal holes or outer retinal holes alone.

Juvenile retinoschisis is a rare and usually X-linked condition that occurs in men. It is congenital, but its manifestations may not be apparent until later in life.

Clinical Presentation: Senile retinoschisis is usually bilateral, with a smooth, domed appearance and most commonly develops inferotemporally (Fig. 25.1.1). There may be non-inflammatory sheathing of retinal blood vessels and retinal 'snowflakes' seen over the inner wall of the schisis cavity. An absolute scotoma is seen on visual field testing, in contrast to the relative scotoma seen in acute rhegmatogenous retinal detachment. Both inner and outer retinal breaks may be seen, but rarely in conjunction. Unlike a retinal detachment, no demarcation line is seen, unless the schisis progresses into a combined detachment.

Patients with juvenile X-linked retinoschisis demonstrate decreased vision associated with macular schisis. More severe loss of vision can occur due to recurrent vitreous hemorrhage, or combined schisis-rhegmatogenous retinal detachment.

OCT Features: Line scans through the area of retinoschisis show a **splitting** of the neurosensory retina, with the split between the inner and outer retinal layers, in contrast to a retinal detachment where the separaration is between the retinal pigment epithelium and the neurosensory retina (Fig. 25.1.2 and 25.1.3). **Hyporeflective spaces** in the nerve fiber layer may represent cystic degeneration.

In juvenile retinoschisis, OCT demonstrates foveal cystic alterations primarily in the outer retinal layers, but eventually the inner retina can be involved as well (Fig. 25.1.4). OCT of the peripheral schisis shows cleavage in the retinal tissue, with bridging retinal elements seen traversing the schisis cavity.

Ancillary Testing: None is needed. Occasionally, visual field testing may be obtained to confirm the presence of an absolute scotoma.

Treatment: Surgery or laser demarcation is indicated only for eyes that develop a concomitant rhegmatogenous retinal detachment in senile retinoschisis.

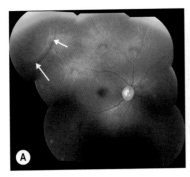
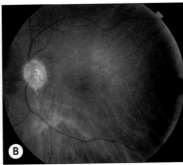

Figure 25.1.1 Fundus photograph of a patient with peripheral retinoschisis (arrows), (A), and one with macular schisis, (B), Note the characteristic cartwheel appearance of the macula.

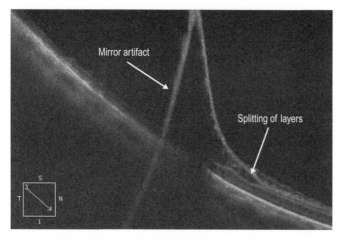

Figure 25.1.2 OCT scan through an area of retinoschisis. Note that the inner and outer retinal layers are separated. Also note the artifactual line seen because the retinoschisis crosses the zero delay line of the OCT scanner.

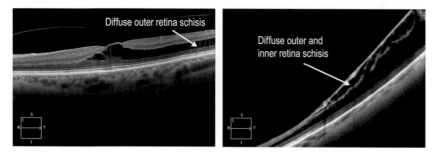

Figure 25.1.4 OCT scan through an area of juvenile retinoschisis. There is schisis with cystic changes at the fovea. There is also peripheral retinoschisis with bands of tissue crossing the schisis cavity.

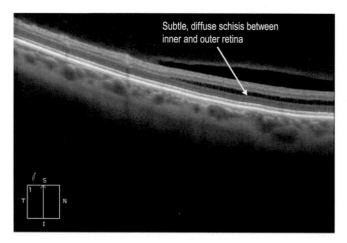

Figure 25.1.3 OCT scan through early retinoschisis showing the development of early cystic changes.

26.1 | Lattice Degeneration

Introduction: Lattice degeneration is a common finding in the peripheral retina. It is characterized by localized retinal thinning with overlying premature vitreous syneresis and traction. This commonly results in atrophic holes, but retinal tears and subsequent retinal detachment are much more uncommon. This condition is estimated to occur in about 8% of the general population, and is more common in moderately myopic individuals. Approximately 40% of eyes with retinal detachments have lattice degeneration.

Clinical Findings: The vast majority of affected patients are asymptomatic with lattice being noted as an incidental finding on a dilated retinal examination. Some patients may complain of photopsias and floaters. Typical lattice consists of sharply demarcated spindle-shaped areas of retinal thinning usually located in the retinal periphery between the equator of the retina and the posterior border of the vitreous base (Fig. 26.1.1). Lattice degeneration occurs more frequently temporally and superiorly in the retina. The retina may be thinned and atrophic. Atrophic holes are the most commonly seen type of retinal break, which typically remain stable, and are rarely associated with retinal detachments. Occasionally, vitreous traction over lattice can cause formation of horseshoe retinal tears which may result in retinal detachment.

OCT Features: **Posterior vitreous separation** may be noted over the area of the lattice. Alternatively, **adherence of the vitreous** over the area of the lattice with separation of vitreous anterior and posterior to the lattice may cause a **U-shaped appearance** to the vitreous (Fig. 26.1.2). This area of U-shaped traction may be associated with **focal retinal detachments** with **hyperreflective areas** within the retina representing disruption of normal cell structure or pigment migration. **Retinal thinning** may also be seen in the area of lattice with the inner retina most severely affected. Areas of **atrophic holes** may be seen within these areas of lattice. **Vitreous membranes** and **cellular aggregates** may also be seen in the vitreous of eyes with lattice degeneration (Figs 26.1.3 and 26.1.4).

Ancillary Testing: Lattice degeneration is best seen with indirect ophthalmoscopy. No ancillary testing is usually needed.

Treatment: Lattice degeneration is usually managed with observation. Based on the low incidence of retinal detachments associated with lattice degeneration and atrophic holes, there is little benefit and even potential harm in prophylactic treatment of lattice and atrophic holes in lattice. However, acute symptomatic retinal holes and tears are treated with prophylactic laser to prevent progression to a retinal detachment.

FIGURE LEGENDS

Figure 26.1.1 Fundus photographs showing lattice degeneration in the mid-peripheral retina (arrows).

Figure 26.1.2 Line scan over the area of lattice degeneration shows vitreous strongly adherent over the area of the lattice (between white arrows) and detached anterior to the lattice. There is traction with a focal tractional detachment over the area of lattice. There is

thinning of the retina especially the inner retina. Also note the thinned choroid that is characteristic of myopia.

Figure 26.1.3 A fibrous band/thickened posterior hyaloid face is seen exerting traction over the area of lattice.

Figure 26.1.4 Debris and cellular aggregates are seen within the vitreous (white arrows).

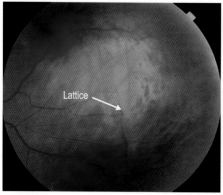
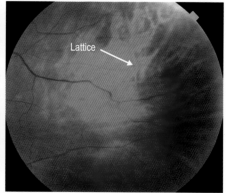

Figure 26.1.1

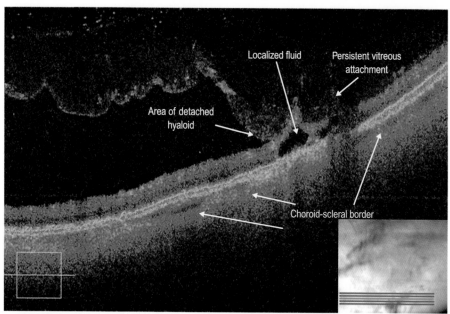

Localized fluid

Persistent vitreous attachment

Area of detached hyaloid

Choroid-scleral border

Figure 26.1.2

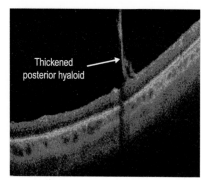

Thickened posterior hyaloid

Figure 26.1.3

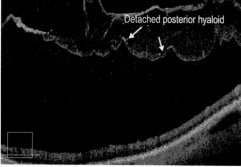

Detached posterior hyaloid

Figure 26.1.4

Index

Page numbers followed by 'f' indicate figures, 't' indicate tables.

Index

W

waterfall effect, 118, 119f
wet age-related macular degeneration, 38–44, 38f–45f

X

X-linked juvenile retinoschisis, 80, 80f–81f

Z

Zeiss Cirrus SD-OCT, 4–6, 5t

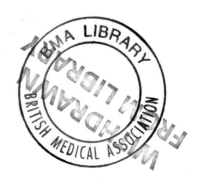